The Ultimate Fit or Fat

Books by Covert Bailey

Fit or Fat?
The Fit-or-Fat Target Diet
The New Fit or Fat
Smart Exercise
The Ultimate Fit or Fat

Books by Covert Bailey and Lea Bishop

Fit-or-Fat Target Recipes
The Fit-or-Fat Woman

Books by Covert Bailey and Ronda Gates

Smart Eating

The Ultimate Fit or Fat

Get in Shape and Stay in Shape
with America's Best-Loved
and Most Effective Fitness Teacher

Covert Bailey

Houghton Mifflin Company
Boston   New York
1999

Covert Bailey Fitness offers programs and materials to help people improve their fitness.

For more information on our fitness and nutrition coaching programs, videotapes, audiotapes, books, and posters:

phone: 1-800-657-7571
e-mail: info@covertbailey.com
Web site: www.covertbailey.com

For information about permission to reproduce selections from this book, write to Permissions, Houghton Mifflin Company, 215 Park Avenue South, New York, New York 10003.

Library of Congress Cataloging-in-Publication Data
Bailey, Covert.
The ultimate fit or fat : Get in shape and stay in shape with America's best-loved and most effective fitness teacher / Covert Bailey.
    p.   cm
    Includes index.
    ISBN 0-618-00204-9
    1. Physical fitness. 2. Aerobic exercises. 3. Reducing exercises. 4. Health. I. Title.
RA781.B215   2000
613.7—dc21   99-40641   CIP

Printed in the United States of America

Book design by Joyce C. Weston

QUM   10 9 8 7 6 5 4 3 2 1

Contents

Excerpt from an Interview with Covert Bailey, August 19, 1999

Q: Your new book . . . is it just a rehash? Or does it have something new to tell us?

A: In this book I have something brand-new, something so radical it will change America. In my little way I'm going to rattle the world. I am going to tackle America's number-one health problem.

Q: By number-one problem, are you referring to heart attacks and strokes?

A: No, heart attacks and strokes are *symptoms* of the problem. Low fitness is the problem. It is the people with unfit arteries, unfit cardiovascular systems, who are vulnerable to heart attacks and strokes. The day is coming when medical insurance will cost half as much for fit people as for fat people. We spend too much time and money on weight-loss programs. People who get fit lose fat without thinking about it — and they get healthy into the bargain. When I put it in that perspective, most people say, "Wow! I've never looked at it that way before!"

Q: Are you claiming your book is going to cure low fitness?

A: Hell, no! People have to cure themselves, but it's hard to take care of yourself when you have no way to measure your progress. If you have to take expensive laboratory tests to find out if you are improving, you tend to lose your incentive. My new book offers methods for monitoring your progress at home. For example, I have a new way to measure body fat so that you can check yourself as often as you want. And I have a brand-new way to measure your own fitness level so that you don't have to wonder how fit you are or how you compare with other people.

Q: Your earlier books talked a lot about aerobic exercise. Is that what *The Ultimate Fit or Fat* is about?
A: Yes, but now we have ways to improve a basic aerobics program, techniques that let you speed up your progress *without* exercising more often or longer.

Q: How do you do that?
A: We used to urge people to do only gentle aerobic exercise. Now we know that you have to add some hard, intense exercise if you want to get fit quickly.

Q: Intense exercise? That sounds scary! Won't people get hurt?
A: They could; that's why most people who talk about how to get fit are afraid to recommend hard exercise. But a big part of this book is about how to add intensity to your exercise *without* getting hurt.

Q: Aren't most exercise teachers still saying, "Take your pulse" and "Be sure you're breathing aerobically"?
A: Either they don't know about the importance of intense exercise or they are afraid of it — intense exercise *has* to be included in a balanced program.

Q: How else has your exercise advice been modified?
A: We now know that weightlifting plays an important role in fitness, and I show you some neat ways to do this at home. People who have never lifted weights like my suggestions because they aren't intimidating, but even macho

types can make good use of my techniques. The book has a whole section on wind sprints, which I never used to recommend for out-of-shape people. But now we know that even fat, unfit people should do wind sprints IF (underline that IF) they learn how to do them right.

Q: **How does one do a wind sprint right?**

A: Aha! Read my book and find out! No, seriously, the reasons why you should do wind sprints, how you should do them, and how they differ for people at various levels of fitness require a rather lengthy explanation. I'm not being flip; it would be irresponsible to throw out a few fast remarks.

Q: **What about diet? Do you talk about that?**

A: Not in this book. I've written two books on diet, *The Fit or Fat Target Diet* and *Smart Eating,* but this new book deals with the underlying problem — fitness. Diet books deal only with a symptom of the problem. My new book explains why people get fat in the first place. It shows you how to change your metabolism — and you can put *that* in capital letters!

Q: **So this is not another diet book?**

A: Right! *The Ultimate Fit or Fat* is not a diet book, but it deals with fat and overweight better than diet books do. The new book tells you how to get fit fast, how to raise your metabolism so you can eat more. And, if that's not enough, how to pass your next physical exam with flying colors.

Q: **What about the baby boomers? They are mostly over fifty now. Is there anything special here for them?**

A: You bet. I'm sixty-seven myself, so I understand the baby boomers' concerns. Getting hurt is a bigger problem with age. But even older people can do hard exercise *if* they learn how to do it right.

Q: **Most people are too lazy. They don't want to exercise.**
A: No! That is not true! People are *not* lazy. If anything, they are rushing around more than ever. The problem is that people are *too busy.* Exercise is only one of their priorities. My book makes it possible to fit exercise into *any* busy schedule.

Q: **If exercise is so good for us, how come doctors don't talk about it?**
A: Because they are too busy taking care of us after we get sick! And they are tired of having people ignore their advice to eat right, keep fit, and quit smoking. The relationship between fitness and health is so obvious that you shouldn't have to have a doctor explain it. For goodness sake, do you want your doctor to hold your hand while you take your daily walk? Don't ask your doctor to be a nanny.

Q: **You have used *The Fit or Fat* in the title of several books. Does *The Ultimate Fit or Fat* mean this is the last of the series?**
A: Yes, it is. The *Fit or Fat* books span twenty years, and although they have been very successful, I have always felt that a key ingredient was missing. In this book nothing is missing. By giving people a way to measure their own fat and their own fitness, *The Ultimate Fit or Fat* pulls together the whole problem of body fat and metabolism. This book gives people the final tools they need to get fit while lowering their fat. At the same time, it should put an end to the diet mania.

1 Covert's Experiment

Let's get a thousand average, ordinary people to help us with an experiment. We'll make sure they are like you and me: men and women, some fit, some fat, some into sports, others not. Let's divide these people into two groups of five hundred, naming one of the groups the "good eaters" and the other the "exercisers."

The good eaters will have the most carefully designed, balanced diet we can devise, BUT they will do little or no exercise. The exercisers will be sloppy in their eating habits, occasionally eating junk food and too much fat and indulging in some weekend pig-outs. BUT they will exercise a lot.

I guarantee you that in twenty years the exercisers will be healthier than the good eaters. They will have had fewer heart attacks, their blood pressure will be lower, and they will have made fewer visits to the doctor's office.

The most obvious difference between the two groups will be the tendency of the good eaters to gain weight, to get fat. Note that I said "tendency." We all know people who are not overweight but who have to eat like birds to stay at their present weight. They have a strong tendency to get fat even if they are not fat.

In contrast, our exercisers tend to stay slim in spite of their dietary excesses. Friends kid them about having a high metabolism. Their fat friends are sure that the exercisers have inherited their tendency toward slimness, that they deserve no credit at all for being slim.

The good eaters continue to search for low-fat, high-vitamin foods while fighting weight gain and putting down the bad dietary habits of the exercisers. I guarantee you that in twenty years, if you talk to any of those five hundred nonexercising, perfect-eating dieters, each one will say, "I just can't understand it! I eat so carefully, but every year I have to eat less and less and still less to keep from gaining weight."

Fit people resist getting fat. This is such an obvious truth that it seems silly to write an entire book on the subject. Yet people cling to the idea that "I got fat because I ate too much, so by golly, I'll get unfat by not eating." Yes, it's true that people get fat when they put more calories into their bodies than can be burned off. But why is it that some people can eat more than 3,000 calories a day without gaining weight while others get fat on 800 calories? Getting fat is much, much more complicated than simply eating too much.

Actually, it's *hard* to get fat by eating too much. Think about it. We've all seen people who eat and eat and never gain weight — they seem to have a hollow leg. In fact, I'm willing to bet that every one of my readers can say, "I used to be that way. I could eat anything I wanted and I never gained weight." We are all born with built-in protective mechanisms that help us resist gaining weight. When we overeat, body temperature rises, "insensible" exercise increases, fat-burning enzyme activity increases, and appetite decreases. Unless we override these protective mechanisms by continuing to eat and eat, our bodies will resist getting fat.

Don't jump to the conclusion that Covert Bailey says you can eat anything you want as long as you exercise. I didn't say that, did I? What I said was, exercise makes you resistant to gaining weight. If we look at our five hundred exercisers

---

TAKE A BREAK!

Here you are, sitting, reading my book (happily, I hope), getting fatter. I have a lot of stuff to tell you, but explaining it will take some time. So, are you just going to sit there doing nothing? Heck, no! Don't say, "Oh! I mustn't do anything until Covert tells me exactly how to do it." You can walk, can't you? Well, put the book down right now, get up, go outside, and walk! Walk in one direction for five minutes, then turn around and walk back for five minutes. Don't try to go super-fast. Just go fast enough that someone watching will think you're on the way to a very important meeting. And you are! You're headed for the most important job you'll ever do — getting fit.

Five minutes out, five minutes back. That's it! Get up, get out, go!!

---

twenty years down the road, we'll find a mixture of fat people and not-fat people. The ones that ate like pigs eventually got fat despite their exercising. The ones who ate sensibly stayed lean. The fat ones in the group will confess, "Yeah, I really overate, but I didn't gain weight for a long, long time." The lean ones will say, "Sure, I overeat now and then, but I don't gain weight unless I *really* pig out."

I won't deny that diet plays a role in whether you get fat or stay lean. But the tendency to get fat is *not* determined by the amount or quality of food you eat.

2 Why People Get Fat

I had a neighbor whose car never seemed to run very well. It was always lurching and coughing down the street. He kept trying one gasoline after another in search of the perfect fuel to make the car run better. Finally I got tired of the noise, and one day, when I couldn't stand it any longer, I recommended a tune-up. He took my advice, and of course after the tune-up his car ran well — on any gasoline.

Think of your body as an automobile. Some of us have sleek race-car bodies with finely tuned engines that require lots of fuel to run well. Others of us are like my neighbor's car, sputtering along with poorly tuned engines that don't seem to run well no matter what kind of fuel we put in them. The engine in your body is muscle. You can feed your muscles the best food and vitamins money can buy, but if they're not tuned up — if they're not exercised — they won't burn up the calories in those foods.

Fat people often blame their weight on recent behavior (like eating too much) instead of looking back through the years for the reason. Getting fat is not a short-term process. It starts with a slowing down of metabolism caused by a decrease in the use of muscle. Obvious fat may not appear for five or even ten years. If you gain weight more easily now than when you were young, it is because your muscles can no longer burn up all the calories you feed them.

The ultimate control of metabolism is exercise. I can't

say that exercise absolutely, without fail, cures obesity, because by eating like a pig, you can overcome the fat-burning benefits of exercise. But exercise can change your metabolism in such a way that you become more and more resistant to gaining weight. Diet books that claim miracle insights into weight control are simply flat-out wrong. **The control mechanism for obesity is not diet, it's muscle metabolism.**

Should you therefore throw out all the diet books and just exercise like crazy? No, you shouldn't. Dieting is quite useful for losing fat temporarily, but it doesn't cure the tendency to get fat easily. We all know people who have lost weight by dieting, only to gain it back when they stop. They lose weight, gain it back, lose some more, and gain again. This pattern is so well known that nutritionists jokingly call it the "rhythm method of girth control." Even if you lose weight on a diet, you aren't fixing the slow metabolism that makes you quickly gain weight again.

Given the phenomenal lack of long-term success inherent

When you put gas in your car, do you ask how much fuel your fenders need? The fat on your body is like the fenders on your car. Do you think your fat fenders are saying, "Feed me! I'm hungry!"? It's not the fenders that need fuel, it's the engine.

If you don't exercise, your muscles atrophy, meaning that your body's engine shrinks. It's as if you'd replaced your big, powerful race-car engine with a smaller, fuel-efficient engine. Now you don't need as much fuel, so that extra food is made into fat fenders!

Some people get so out of shape that it's as if they'd replaced their car engine with a lawn mower — and they're towing a trailer!!

in most weight-loss diets, you'd think people wouldn't be suckered into trying them again and again. People who fall for this con game are like compulsive gamblers, sure that they've found the secret for beating the odds. If you play the weight-loss game by dieting, you may get short-term results, but you won't win in the end. You're going up against the house — metabolism — hopelessly trying for a big win — fast weight loss — against all the odds. Diets are not the answer because they don't improve metabolism. The only way to improve metabolism is to exercise.

I wish I could get fat people to stay away from diet books and friends who claim to have lost a lot of weight. Instead, they should seek out skinny creatures and ask, "How do you stay so skinny? What do you do?" They should watch how these creatures live instead of watching what they eat. A fat person should ask a fox, a deer, or even the family dog how he stays so skinny. These animals stay thin because they exercise, exercise, exercise, not because they diet.

3   Never Say Diet

The fat person says, "I just can't lose weight." But when you ask the typical fat person if he has ever lost weight on a diet, he will tell you of the thirty pounds he lost on this diet and the twenty pounds he lost on that one. In fact, many of the people I have interviewed have lost a thousand pounds over the years! Clearly, losing weight was not their problem at all. Not only do they lose weight very easily, they lose on practically every diet they try.

Yes, diets help people lose weight, but losing weight is not the basic problem. The problem is — gaining weight! Fat people gain weight easily and quickly, so before long they have more fat than they have just lost.

Suppose you had a broken leg and your doctor treated it simply with a shot of painkiller and sent you home. When the painkiller wore off, you would realize the doctor hadn't treated the basic problem. He should have set your leg and put it in a cast. When you diet away your fat, you aren't treating the real problem. After you finish the diet, you may have lost some fat, but you haven't lost your tendency to get fat. You haven't corrected the problem of what makes you gain weight more easily than other people do.

> Fat people who are constantly dieting should worry less about how to lose weight. Instead they should ask themselves, "Why do I gain weight so easily?"

On one of my television appearances the host handed me a book and asked, "What do you think of this new diet book?" Well, I didn't like being put on the spot like that. It wasn't fair to ask me to analyze a book I'd never seen before. But after looking at it for about five seconds I said, "This diet book is a total rip-off."

Later, my staff wanted to know how I had the nerve to say that after only glancing at the book. It was easy. All I had to do was look at the cover, which claimed "Guaranteed permanent weight loss with no exercise." No way, absolutely impossible! The book may have had some good things to say, but that one statement condemned it. If I handed you a five-dollar bill that said "counterfeit" in one corner, you wouldn't take it. I might say, "Why not? It only says counterfeit in one place." Well, counterfeit is counterfeit! Any diet book that claims permanent weight loss *without* exercise is counterfeit!

When a *fit* person eats 1,000 calories, all of them get burned, wasted, used up. When a *fat* person eats 1,000 calories, only some of them are used up, while the remainder are converted to fat. If the fat person adjusts his diet so he eats fewer calories, his body learns to function on still fewer. Again he is left with extra calories that will be stored as fat.

The fat person needs to retrain his body so that it burns up ALL the calories it gets, storing none as fat. Yes, he may need a diet at the start to help lose excess fat. But long-term weight control requires a change in body chemistry so he won't get fat all over again. I'm sure you know what I'm going to recommend. Exercise is the ONLY WAY to change your metabolism so that your body converts fewer calories to fat. In later chapters I'm going to show you some fast and efficient ways to exercise. I have some neat tricks and shortcuts to make it fun.

But first, how fat should you be?

4 Body Fat Percentage — What's Normal?

There's a lot of nitpicking going on concerning "correct" body fat percentages. Everyone seems to have a different "correct" number. Doctors tell us that 120/80 is normal blood pressure, but they know that a little deviation to either side of normal is okay. If your blood pressure is a little high, let's say 125/85, it doesn't mean you are going to die tomorrow. It is just a warning sign that something is a little off, that you need to monitor your blood pressure.

Similarly, we believe that men should try to keep their body fat to 15 percent or less. A man with 19 percent body fat isn't going to die tomorrow. But that much body fat suggests that fat is slowly settling into his arteries. He is at risk for future heart attacks, strokes, and kidney disease. He isn't sick, but he may be more vulnerable to illnesses.

For women, we recommend no more than 22 percent fat. If a woman's fat percentage gets a little higher than this, say 26 percent, she's probably still quite active and living a good life. It's just that now she has to struggle more to keep from gaining weight, and she, too, is more at risk for heart disease, diabetes, and other fat-related problems.

The numbers 15 percent for men and 22 percent for women are not carved in stone, any more than 98.6 degrees is for body temperature or 120/80 for blood pressure. There are, for example, ethnic differences; Asians fare well with slightly higher percentages of fat, while blacks should maintain slightly lower levels.

So the 15 percent fat for men and 22 percent for women, which I will use throughout the rest of this book, are guidelines, not laws; they help us to derive other useful information. These numbers are indicators of health, just as 120/80 is for blood pressure. Above and below those percentages we begin to ask questions about your body.

Men should be no more than 15 percent fat.
Women should be no more than 22 percent fat.

Good athletes usually have much lower fat percentages. Lean male cross-country runners are often as low as 7 percent, and female runners may be 14 percent. Gymnasts, with their highly muscled bodies, have even lower fat, 3–5 percent for men and 9–13 percent for women. Ten or fifteen years ago, when professional football teams were first measured for fat, the heavyweight linemen averaged about 17 percent and the faster-moving quarterbacks about 10 percent. The linemen, you notice, were slightly over our theoretical 15 percent; a little extra fat meant extra weight, which was presumably an advantage. Today those linemen would be kicked off the team for being too fat. College athletes may get away with slightly higher fat levels, but on a professional football team the "front four" players all have less than 10 percent fat inside three-hundred-pound bodies! If you see one of these men running toward you — step aside!

Of the thousands of people we have measured,

The average man is 22 percent fat.
The average woman is 32 percent fat.

In other words, most men and women are 7 to 10 percent above healthful fat levels. Don't confuse "average" with

Body Fat Percentages (Data Obtained from Underwater Immersion Testing)

	Men (%)	Women (%)
Lowest I've tested	1	6
Top Athletes	2–12	10–18
Gymnasts	5	10
Rock climbers	5	10
Runners	7	14
Body builders	10	16
Aerobic dance instructors	12	18
Cyclists	13	20
Swimmers	14	22
Healthy*	15 max.	22 max.
Average	22	32
Highest I've tested	55	68

* The percentages, 15 percent for men and 22 percent for women, are the *highest* a person should have to be healthy.

"healthy." To be five or ten pounds overweight may seem normal, and all your slightly overweight friends may look normal, but that doesn't mean they are healthy. Those friends are *average*, not healthy.

The higher fat level in women, even those who are a healthful 22 percent, may partially explain the greater incidence of obesity in women than men. Since women have more fat to start with, it's easier for them to get fatter. Why are women fatter? The obvious answer is hormones. At puberty, boys and girls have approximately the same per-

> If a woman is fat I have a lot of sympathy for her, because her hormones, her lower muscle mass, and having children all contribute to her fat.
> A man has no excuse for being fat. A fat man has nothing to blame except overeating and laziness.

centage of fat, around 14–17 percent. Then, when the female and male hormones kick in, big changes occur. Male hormones induce muscle growth while suppressing the storage of fat. Female hormones stimulate the deposition of fat. (Most likely this is a safety mechanism so that a pregnant woman will have extra fat to nourish her baby, even if she can't get enough calories to feed herself properly.) The boys get progressively leaner while the girls get progressively fatter. A healthy teenage boy is about 10–12 percent fat, while his healthy, fit girlfriend is 20–22 percent.

A less obvious reason why women are fatter is that with puberty, girls "grow up," putting aside tomboy games for pretty dresses and makeup. Boys, if anything, do just the opposite, getting even more heavily involved in sports. Now I'll admit that times are changing and that girls are learning how to be both pretty AND fit, but in the past women tended to exercise less than men.

When we put those two facts together — women's hormones make them fatter and women tend to exercise less than men — you can see why women are fatter than men and have more trouble getting rid of the fat. And after a woman has a baby, it's even harder for her to lose weight.

At this point, the question of body type often arises. You may reason that 15 percent and 22 percent are normal for mesomorphs, but shouldn't ectomorphs, the "natural skinnys," have less fat than that? And shouldn't the endomorphs, the "natural fatsos," have more? My answer is an emphatic

I've become pretty good at estimating body fat by gripping a person's arm and squeezing the waist. Low-fat people have solid arms and waistlines. When you ask them to "tighten up," they can make their arm or waist rock-hard. As a person becomes more and more out of shape and the muscles fill up with fat, the arms and waistline become softer and softer. I remember a tall, thin young woman I tested who had never exercised a day in her life. I gripped her arm and said, "Tighten up, Susie."

"Okay!" she said obligingly. I waited a few seconds, but her arm felt as soft as ever.

"Tighten up, Susie," I repeated.

"I am, I am!" she grunted, her face red from the effort.

This woman was so out of shape and her muscles were so soft that no amount of flexing made them harder. She *looked* thin on the outside, but she was fat on the inside.

no! All men should strive for 15 percent maximum fat, and all women should aim for 22 percent maximum fat. A 200-pound man can carry 30 pounds of fat, which is 15 percent of his weight. A 160-pound man should carry only 24 pounds of fat, which is also 15 percent of his weight. If a man has large bones and a lot of muscle, he can carry more fat without exceeding the 15 percent. He may weigh more than another man who is the same height and has lighter bones, but they both should shoot for 15 percent fat or less.

I have seen people who might have been considered natural fatsos who were able to lower their fat level to a point where they didn't fit the endomorph label anymore. But what is even more astonishing is to find that many ectomorphs, who appear quite thin, even skinny, have an unexpectedly high percentage of fat.

Rather than using the terms mesomorph, ectomorph, and

endomorph to describe apparent differences in body type, I prefer to discard them completely in favor of fat percentages.

People often ask if it's okay to be a little fatter as you get older. I'll admit that it's much harder for older people to keep their fat percentage low. Many older people don't exercise as vigorously as they did when they were young. They're more likely to have "down" time because of an injury or illness, and recovery takes longer. And as one ages, some bone and muscle are lost, so the nonfat part of the body shrinks. Here again, women are behind the eight ball. Most men don't experience muscle and bone loss until they are into their seventies, while women usually experience it ten to fifteen years earlier. Additionally, menopause speeds up bone loss. Women have to decide whether to take an estrogen replacement — which tends to add more fat — or risk a faster and greater diminishment of bone density.

Given all this, *should* older men and women have higher fat percentages? The simple answer is NO! I'll discuss my reasons for saying no in Chapter 6, "Lean Body Mass and Correct Weight." Right now let's figure out how fat YOU are.

People ask, "Can you be zero percent fat?" Well, the brain is made of fat ... If you got to zero percent fat the only profession you could go into would be politics!

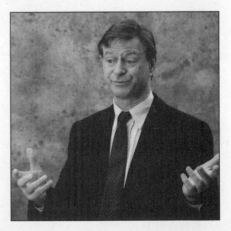

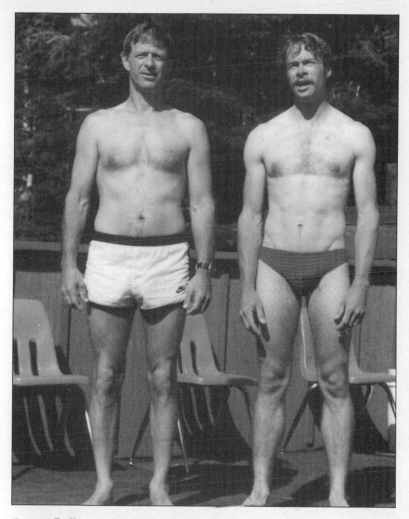

Covert Bailey and Bob Pinckney, 1986
Bob was my right-hand man for years. I'm 13 percent fat in this picture (and fifty-four years old), so I'm pretty proud of myself. But you can see a little bit of fat starting to accumulate around my belly.

Bob was an avid rock climber. Like gymnasts, rock climbers get very low in fat and have great upper body musculature. Bob, at thirty-four years old, has only 6 percent body fat!

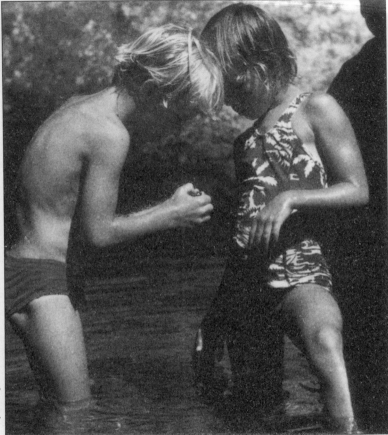

Sally Bailey

Christina and Grant Bailey, 1976

I first tested my children for body fat when Grant was six years old and Christina was five. I continued to test them and their friends throughout their teenage years and into adulthood. We learned that healthy, active children — both boys and girls — generally have the same amount of body fat, about 15 percent. Once they hit puberty, however, big changes occur. When testosterone kicks in, body fat in the boys drops as they "muscle up"; meanwhile, estrogen production in the girls increases body fat. By the time they are twenty, healthy, active boys are usually 12–15 percent fat, and healthy, active girls are 18–22 percent fat.

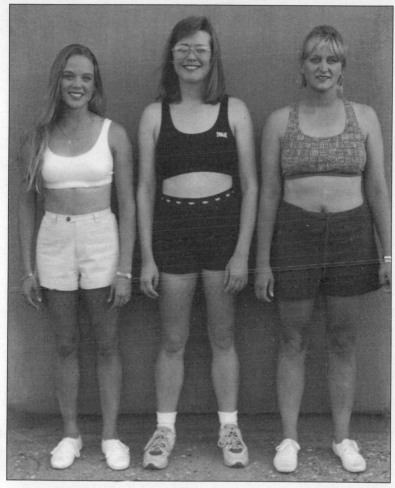

Matt Wilson

One of these women is 22 percent fat. Can you guess which one?

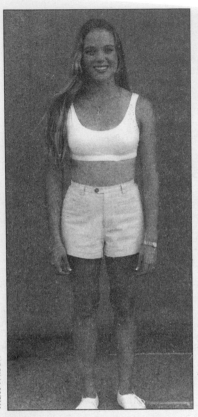

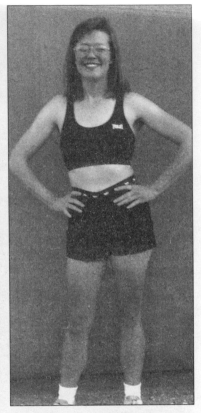

Matt Wilson

Teresa, 17 percent fat, aerobics instructor
Teresa teaches three one-hour aerobics classes a day, five days a week. In addition she fills her weekends with hard skiing in the winter and competition tennis in the summer. That's a lot of exercise, and her low body fat percentage reflects it. Most women, with less time for exercise, won't get below 22 percent fat.

Bonnie, 22 percent fat
Bonnie, who is thirty years old, jogs twenty to thirty minutes three days a week, does mild upper-body weightlifting, and loves to go on bicycle treks on weekends. She gets lots of exercise, but she is quite relaxed and not competitive about it. At 22 percent fat, she's at the "ideal" healthful fat percentage for women. Her weight doesn't fluctuate very much, and she can eat pretty much what she wants without gaining.

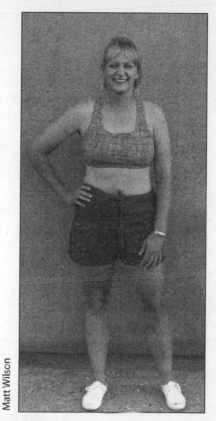

Matt Wilson

Ginger, 32 percent fat

Ginger is a good example of the "average" woman. At 32 percent fat, she's about twenty pounds overweight. Like most overfat people, she tends to gain weight easily if she doesn't watch her diet all the time. She has two young children and a gorgeous garden she loves to work in. What with caring for her children and her garden, she's busy all the time. Ginger can't understand why she doesn't lose weight. The problem, I told her, is that she's confusing work with exercise. Even though she's busy all the time, she does no sustained fat-reducing aerobic exercise.

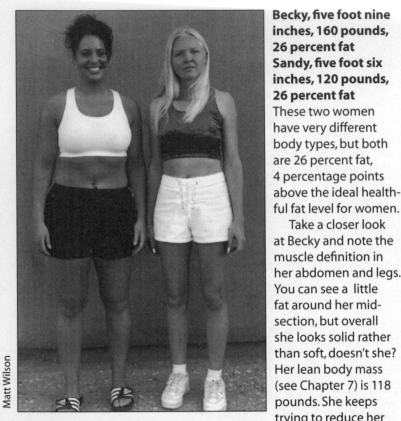

Matt Wilson

Becky, five foot nine inches, 160 pounds, 26 percent fat
Sandy, five foot six inches, 120 pounds, 26 percent fat
These two women have very different body types, but both are 26 percent fat, 4 percentage points above the ideal healthful fat level for women.

Take a closer look at Becky and note the muscle definition in her abdomen and legs. You can see a little fat around her midsection, but overall she looks solid rather than soft, doesn't she? Her lean body mass (see Chapter 7) is 118 pounds. She keeps trying to reduce her weight to 135, but she has so much bone and muscle she should weigh more than that. I told her she would be 22 percent fat if she got down to 151 pounds. Now you know why she's smiling!

Sandy has fewer pounds of fat than Becky, but she also has fewer pounds of bone and muscle to carry her fat. Even though she is slimmer and smaller, her fat percentage is the same as Becky's. Sandy is thirty-four and has four children. She has had a hysterectomy and is now on hormone replacement therapy. Even though she exercises regularly and eats low-fat foods, her fat level is higher than the ideal because of childbearing and hormone replacement. For Sandy, I consider 28 percent fat to be healthful and would not recommend that she try to lower it.

It is easy to see which man is the fattest — but take a guess at which one is the lowest in fat.

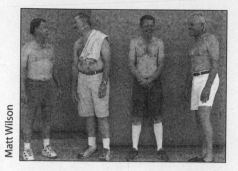

Matt Wilson

Robert, 23 percent fat
Steve, 28 percent fat

Both of these men are in their fifties. Robert is the "average" man. He's 23 percent fat and is carrying 175 pounds on his six-foot frame. A very busy physician, he is currently building his own home and coaching boy's soccer on the weekends. Like Ginger, he works all the time yet never does any real exercise. He's gotten fat doing all that "busywork."

Steve is 28 percent fat, much too high for good health. I sometimes call men who are this high in fat "walking heart attacks." He needs to start exercising and cutting fat out of his diet NOW! Steve is a big

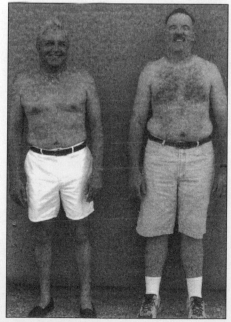

Matt Wilson

man — six foot two, weighing 245 pounds. He has a huge lean body mass, 175 pounds, which is as much lean weight as Robert has total weight. With that much lean, Steve's correct weight would be 210 pounds. Like Becky, he was very pleased to learn this, because he thought he should weigh 180. With the more realistic goal of 210, Steve started a two-mile-a-day walking/jogging program, and he says he'll never eat butter, margarine, or any other greasy food topping again.

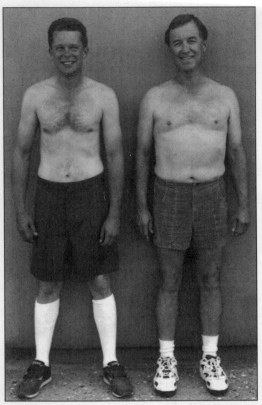

Matt Wilson

Matt, 21 percent fat
Don, 16 percent fat
Matt will surprise
you. He looks thin, but
he's actually 21 per-
cent fat. You can't see
any obvious fat, but
he *feels* soft. The mus-
cles in his arms and
abdomen are spongy
to the grip. He thinks
he looks too thin,
his mother thinks he
looks too thin, and his
friends tell him to
"fatten up." So that's
exactly what he has
done. Matt eats lots of
high-fat foods, think-
ing he'll look heftier.
What he really needs
to do is *muscle* up.
He needs to exercise
aerobically to burn
the fat out of his mus-
cles and then add weightlifting to bulk up his muscles.

Don may look fatter, but in fact most of his girth is bone and muscle. He is only 16 percent fat, quite a bit lower than Matt. (For good
health, men should be 15 percent fat.) He's sixty years old, and his
main activity is playing tennis one or two hours a day. Tennis isn't the
most *efficient* way to burn fat, but because Don does so much of it,
he has managed to keep his fat low. Don has another advantage in
that he was a high school wrestler. Ex-athletes tend to have an easier
time maintaining low fat throughout their lives. Let that be a lesson to
the younger people reading this book: get fit now so you won't have
to fight fat later.

5 How to Measure Your Body Fat

There are many ways to measure body fat, but by far the most precise method is based on how well you float. In our clinic we use an underwater immersion test, weighing people on a hanging scale while they are completely immersed. The more readily they sink, the leaner they are. The more fat they have, the more they tend to float and the less they weigh underwater.

The underwater immersion test is time-consuming, takes up lots of laboratory space, and is scary for many people, so most testing facilities use less accurate but more convenient methods. Most techniques measure the fat just beneath the skin, on the assumption that the amount of subcutaneous fat increases as total body fat increases. When you consider all the places inside the body where fat can accumulate, such as around the intestines and inside muscles, it's hard to believe that measuring skin fat would reflect total body fat, but we have measured people's fat both underwater and with the skin test for years and, using our formula, subcutaneous fat measurements are amazingly accurate.

Covert Bailey's Tape-Measure Formula

Women Thirty Years and Younger

hips + (.80 × thigh) − (2 × calf) − wrist = % body fat

Example: hips = 36″; thigh = 21″; calf = 12″, wrist = 5³/₄″.

36 + (.80 × 21 = 16.80) − (2 × 12 = 24) − 5.75 = 23% body fat

Women over Thirty

hips + thigh − (2 × calf) − wrist = % body fat

Example: hips = 39″; thigh = 23″; calf = 13¹/₂″; wrist = 6″.

39 + 23 − (2 × 13.5 = 27) − 6 = 29% body fat

Men Thirty Years and Younger

waist + (¹/₂ hips) − (3 × forearm) − wrist = % body fat

Example: waist = 34″; hips = 36″; forearm = 11″; wrist = 7″.

34 + (¹/₂ × 36 = 18) − (3 × 11 = 33) − 7 = 12% body fat

Men over Thirty

waist + (¹/₂ hips) − (2.7 × forearm) − wrist = % body fat

Example: waist = 40″; hips = 40″; forearm = 10³/₄″; wrist = 7″.

40 + (¹/₂ × 40 = 20) − (2.7 × 10.75 = 29.0) − 7 = 24% body fat

Where to Measure

Use a cloth tape, one that hasn't gotten stretched out.

Waist. Stand up straight but don't suck in your stomach; be relaxed. Measure your waist at the greatest circumference. Men sometimes have trouble with this measurement.

It can vary by five inches quite easily. For example, Covert gets:

1. Maximum suck-in of gut   32 inches
2. Relaxed but still consciously sucking in   33 inches
3. Comfortable, but still self-conscious/ unconscious sucking in   34 inches
4. Probably the way he usually is when no one else is around   35 inches
5. Blown out, deliberately exaggerated belly   38 inches

Please play around with the measurements a little. Get all five and run them through the formula; you'll find there's quite a variation. You may be tempted to use the results of 1, 2, or 3, but the results of 4 are the most accurate.

Hips. People sometimes take this measurement incorrectly by placing the tape too high. You should wrap it around your hips and your buttocks. Stand with your feet about four inches apart and measure the greatest circumference.

For the following measurements, use your dominant side (right-handed people measure the right; left-handed people measure the left).

Thigh. Stand with your feet about twelve inches apart; measure the upper thigh at the widest part.

Calf. Distribute your weight evenly on both feet; measure the calf at the widest part, about midway between the knee and the ankle.

Forearm. Clench your fist so that your forearm is flexed; measure at the widest part between the wrist and elbow.

Wrist. Measure just above the bony protuberance (toward the hand).

I've found that for most men and women our tape-measure test is within 2 percent of the "real thing," that is, the immersion test. If a man tests at 17 percent in water, the tape-measure test will give a number between 15 and 19 percent.

For some people, however, the results of the immersion test are quite different from those of the tape-measure test. Very, very fit people get numbers 3–5 percent *higher* on the tape-measure test compared to water immersion because they have, in a sense, "cleaned out" their intramuscular fat, so they are lower in body fat than the tape measure indicates. (See the chart "How Fit Are You?" in Chapter 14 for more on this subject.)

Conversely, if a person is skinny but not fit, the tape-measure test yields a number 3–5 percent *lower* than the immersion test. Unfit skinny people have more than the usual amount of fat inside their muscles. They may not look fat on the outside, and the tape-measure test may say they're normal, but the underwater immersion results would say, "Uh-uh, your muscles are *greasy* on the inside!"

Please, please, don't skip this body fat test. We have tested body fat for years, experimenting with every formula and every gizmo we could find. We concluded early on that the underwater immersion test was the best, and we still think so. But I made the same mistake many medical professionals make. I thought that underwater weighing, especially if done in my clinic, was the *only* accurate way to test body fat. Accuracy was the most important thing, I thought. Suppose, however, that we determined in our clinic that your fat percentage was 18.6 percent. You would go home quite impressed, I hope. But two months later that number might not be accurate at all. If you lost or gained weight, you'd want

---

> ### TIME FOR ANOTHER BREAK!
> Go for another ten-minute walk, but take a different direction this time. If you want to be more adventuresome, you can improve your balance and coordination by adding thirty-second intervals of "silly stuff," like walking sideways or backward or on your tiptoes. When I was writing this book, I took ten-minute breaks. Every hour or two I'd go outdoors and walk briskly for three or four minutes. Then I'd launch into a legs-bent Groucho Marx routine. Or I'd do a sideways polka. Sometimes I'd just zig and zag across the road. Neighbors watching would yawn and say, "Covert must be writing another book." If your neighbors inquire about your antics, tell them, "I'm reading Covert's book!"

to know if your fat percentage had changed. Even if your weight *hadn't* changed, there might be other reasons to check your body fat. What if you had been on a radical diet? Or been sick?

It's just not practical to have an immersion test every time you want to check your body fat. The tape-measure test is quite accurate, it puts you in control, it can be done frequently, and it costs nothing.

The tape-measure test doesn't involve computers with impressive printouts or machines with blinking lights, but you should not underrate its value. Being able to monitor yourself at any time — summer, winter, before and after a vacation, before and after a diet — is a far more powerful tool than fancy equipment used once a year. You can spend lots of dollars at high-tech clinics getting high-tech tests, but nothing beats self-measurement.

COVERT BAILEY'S HOME IMMERSION TEST*

For fun, I've devised a fat test that can be done in a swimming pool.

Float on your back in the pool. Even if this is easy for you, it is best to get a friend to help by lifting very lightly under the small of your back. Relax completely, lowering your head until your ears are almost under water; then put your arms out to the sides and slightly above your head. Relax and breathe normally. Once you are comfortable, have your friend gradually release all assistance.

If you can stay afloat in this position, breathing shallowly, you are at 20 –25 percent fat, a proper fat level for a woman, but too high for a man.

On the other hand, if you are breathing shallowly but you slowly sink, you have 14 –18 percent fat, the range for healthy men and very low for women.

If you take a huge lungful of air and hold it, and you still sink, you are below 13 percent fat, like most athletes.

Now try this. Air, like fat, keeps you afloat. Exhale completely; that is, blow out all your air. If you stay afloat, you are being buoyed up by more than 25 percent body fat — you are probably over 28 percent fat.

If you can float while holding a gin and tonic in one hand and balancing a five-pound book on your stomach with the other hand, you are in big trouble!

*These numbers are only approximate, because your floatability is also affected by age, lung volume, and water temperature. The real immersion test isn't as simple as it sounds and can't be done accurately at home.

6 Lean Body Mass and Correct Weight

In calculating correct weight, we start with a person's lean body mass (LBM) rather than age, height, or body type. The weight tables that your physician used to use were useful when nothing better was available, but it is clear now that they can be off by twenty to thirty pounds. It is possible to be overweight according to the charts yet be very low in fat. And the reverse is true. We have measured many skinny people who are underweight according to the charts but overfat. They don't look fat but they are, because their muscles are loaded with it.

Lean body mass is the weight of the nonfat part of the body. Although LBM includes the organs, blood, and water, the main components are bone and muscle. If we know how much lean body mass you have, we can determine your ideal weight. A person with a large LBM has large bones and muscles, and we would project a greater weight for that person than for someone of the same height who has thin bones and small muscles.

Let's take as an example a man at four different times in his life. When he is a twenty-year-old college student involved in wrestling, gymnastics, and weightlifting, lots of muscle has been added to his frame, making his lean body mass 145 pounds. He can carry 25 pounds of fat while weighing 170 pounds.

A Man at 15 Percent Fat*

Age	Total weight (lbs.)	Fat (lbs.)	LBM (lbs.)	Activity
20	170	25	145	Wrestling
38	162	24	138	Running
45	135	20	115	Prison camp
70	155	23	132	Covert's program

*Maintaining 15% body fat despite changes in muscle mass as activities change.

At thirty-eight, he is a businessman whose only real physical activity beyond weekend skiing and some golf is running. The running keeps him lean and healthy, but it is not a sport that packs on much muscle. In fact, since running doesn't use upper-body muscle, he will actually lose some of it. So now he has only 138 pounds of lean body mass. He shouldn't carry more than 24 pounds of fat and shouldn't exceed 162 pounds. His body adapts beautifully to its new role. Obviously, a runner doesn't need the upper-body musculature of a gymnast. As muscle mass decreases, total weight should decrease also.

Let's take a third situation. Suppose our man, now in his forties, undergoes some kind of extreme deprivation, such as two years of near starvation in a prison camp or a debilitating disease. He will lose much fat and much muscle. At the end of such hardship, he will be haggard and thin. His wife, and probably his physician, will want to fatten him up. I emphatically disagree with that approach. If his lean mass has dropped to 115 pounds, he should not carry more than 20 pounds of fat and shouldn't weigh more than 135. The only healthful recourse for such an individual is to replace the lost

> ### OLD PEOPLE
>
> Okay, you're old. Or you think you're old. Certainly your children think you're old. So what should you do differently from everybody else, and will this book help you do it? Well, I'm sixty-seven, and to tell you the truth, I am slowing down a bit. I feel stiff in the morning, my joints sometimes ache, and I get tired more easily.
>
> Yes, I know what it's like to get old. But what should I do about it? Give up? Buy a recliner? Not me, and I hope not you. Old, to me, means getting smarter, getting wiser. It means learning how to exercise without getting hurt. It means learning to play again. Remember when we were kids? All we wanted to do was play, but the grownups made us go to school, study, and get a job. And we forgot how to play! The richest part of getting older is learning how to play all over again.
>
> As you read this book, don't look for special sections about old people. Yes, there are special considerations, and I touch on them throughout the book. But use your smarts. Study my principles, then modify them for an older body. So read on — what follows is for everyone. Let's show the kids what fun it is to get old!

muscle, adding fat only to maintain 15 percent. If he eats to add weight, he will add only *fat*, even though he may still appear thin.

The effects of old age can mimic the effects of hardship. Suppose our man hasn't spent time in a prison camp as described but has lived a good healthy life into his seventies. He's still quite active, but the 145-pound lean body mass he had as a teenager has now dropped to 132 pounds. He's not sick, he's not calorie-deprived, he's simply aging, so his bones are more porous and his muscles not quite so dense. Since his lean mass is smaller, he needs to reduce his *total* weight so that once again no more than 15 percent of it is fat. Women have less bone and muscle mass to begin with and they lose it much earlier than men; at fifty or sixty they experience the loss of lean mass that men face at sixty or seventy.

> Older men and women should shoot for 15 percent (men) and 22 percent body fat (women). BUT! In order to do that, most will have to DECREASE their total body weight.

In Chapter 4, we asked whether older people should be allowed to have a higher fat percentage. My answer was *no*, they should not. Older people should *not* gain weight as they age; instead, they need to gradually decrease their weight over the years so that they can maintain a healthful level of body fat. As lean body mass decreases, so too should total body weight.

There is an exception. Just like the twelve-year-old girl who after puberty has a higher percentage of fat, an older

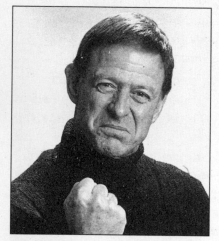

woman taking postmenopausal hormones (or, for that matter, a younger woman taking birth control pills) *should* be slightly higher in body fat. Women taking postmenopausal hormones should aim for 25–30 percent body fat; women taking birth control pills should aim for 23–26 percent body fat.

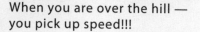

When you are over the hill — you pick up speed!!!

7 Fat Versus Lean — What's Healthy?

After testing thousands of men and women in our clinic, we realized that men and women carry practically the same amount of fat. Most of us have around twenty-five pounds of fat if we're *healthy* and forty or fifty pounds if we're *average*. It doesn't matter whether we're male or female. The *pounds of fat* we carry are about the same.

But let's not talk about fat anymore. Let's drop the fat talk and instead talk about what's left, the lean part of our bodies. Now we see a big difference between men and women. Men have anywhere from twenty to forty more pounds of lean body mass, mainly muscle and bone, than women. And it's the amount of lean we have, not the amount of fat, that determines how easily we gain or lose weight. It doesn't seem fair, but because women have considerably less lean than men, they not only gain weight more easily but it's also more difficult for them to lose the weight they gain.

When I talk about "lean" I am thinking mostly about muscle, because that's the part that can be changed. Technically, lean body mass includes bones and other soft tissue, but those parts don't have high metabolisms and can't be changed very easily. Muscle, on the other hand, can be increased or decreased and can be trained to burn fat.

The muscle on your body is similar to the engine in your car. It's the part of your body that uses the most calories. Your hair doesn't need calories, your fingernails don't need calories. Just picture a woman with long beautiful hair saying, "Oh! I must eat more because I have such long hair!" Similarly, you don't need to send calories to your fat. Fat IS calories. Muscle, the underlying engine, burns most of the calories you eat. Because men's engines are considerably bigger than women's, they can eat more without gaining weight. And, if they do gain weight, their bigger engines burn off the excess fat more readily than a woman's smaller engine.

While it's fun to talk about how much fat we have, the significant number is — how much lean do we have? To find out, however, we have to talk about fat again. We have to first determine how many *pounds of fat* we have.

HOW MANY POUNDS OF FAT DO YOU HAVE?

Using the *body fat percentage* you got from Covert Bailey's Tape-Measure Formula in Chapter 4:

(total weight) × (percent body fat) = pounds of fat

For example, Jim is a healthy 15 percent fat and weighs 170 pounds:

170 × .15 = 25 pounds of fat

I remember Jim. He looked lean, fit, and rugged, yet somewhere, slathered throughout his body, were twenty-five pounds of fat. Let's take a moment to think about that. Suppose his wife asked him to get some butter at the supermarket. "Sure, honey, how much do you need?" Oh, just — twenty-five pounds! Imagine twenty-five pounds of butter stacked up in a grocery cart. You'd have trouble putting it all away in the refrigerator. Where in the world does twenty-five pounds of fat go in your body? And that's the amount we find in healthy people. Just imagine the forty or fifty pounds of fat packed on the average man or woman.

But I said we wouldn't talk about fat anymore. Instead, let's find out how much of you is high-powered, calorie-burning engine.

HOW MUCH LEAN DO YOU HAVE?

total weight – pounds of fat = lean body mass
Jim, from the previous example, is 15 percent fat, weighs 170 pounds, and has 25 pounds of fat:

170 – 25 = 145 pounds of lean body mass

Let's get Jim's butter-loving wife into the picture and compare the two:

	Percent body fat	Weight (lbs.)	Pounds of fat	Pounds of lean
Jim	15	170	25	145
Bonnie	22	120	26	94

Both Jim and Bonnie have healthful amounts of fat, but look at the difference between their amounts of lean. Jim has fifty more pounds of lean fat-burning potential than his wife.

After measuring the lean body mass of about ten thousand people, we derived the chart below. We excluded from the chart people who were either very fat or extremely skinny. Note that lean body mass for men is considerably greater than for women even when they are the same height. Since it's the muscle in lean body mass that burns calories, men get to eat a lot more without gaining weight.

Lean Body Mass of Men with 15% Fat and Women with 22% Fat*

Height	Men (lbs.)	Women (lbs.)
5'0"		74–86
5'1"		76–90
5'2"		78–94
5'3"	94–115	82–98
5'4"	99–119	83–100
5'5"	106–125	87–105
5'6"	115–132	90–111
5'7"	119–137	94–117
5'8"	125–140	98–122
5'9"	131–149	103–127
5'10"	139–157	109–129
5'11"	144–166	113–136
6'0"	149–179	117–140
6'1"	153–191	
6'2"	157–199	
6'3"	161–204	
6'4"	166–212	

*These lean body mass numbers were compiled from tests of active men and women who were close to the ideal body fat percentages.

SKINNY FATS AND HEAVY LEAN GUYS

I kept a straight face when Alice dragged her daughter to my clinic, but inside I was smiling. "You've got to do something to help Trish lose weight!" Alice implored. "She already weighs twenty pounds more than me and she's only fifteen years old!"

Trish looks solid as a rock, I thought to myself. I suggested we test her body fat to see how much she should weigh, and, just for the fun of it, test her mother as well. Alice was happy to be tested. At thirty-eight, she had maintained her high school weight with careful dieting for the past twenty years. She looked trim — but to me she also looked soft.

> Big people are not always fat.
> Skinny people are not always lean.

Sure enough, when we did the body fat test, Alice was overfat. At 32 percent, she looked slender, but she was fat inside. Over the years, fat had seeped in and around her underexercised muscles, giving them the appearance of the marbling we see in tender, high-fat steaks. Her fat had piled up while her muscles had atrophied from disuse. In a sense, fat had replaced muscle, so she hadn't gained weight. She was getting fatter but not heavier. But muscles can hold only so much fat! Eventually fat is deposited outside of muscle, under the skin. This subcutaneous fat doesn't replace anything; it is simply an addition, so the person's weight begins to climb. It would be only a matter of time before Alice's marbled muscles refused to hide any more fat and it would "spill over" under her skin; she would gain weight.

Alice's daughter, on the other hand, was a "lean heavy gal." Trish, who was captain of her soccer team, skied or hiked with her brothers on the weekends and ran a couple of miles a day just for fun. At five foot five inches, she weighed 140 pounds. She thought she was overweight, and her mother thought she was overweight, but by looking at Trish's firm muscles I knew they were both wrong. The body fat test confirmed it. Trish was only 16 percent fat!

Although Trish weighed 140 pounds, she looked as if she weighed 125; her lean muscles gave her a slim, well-toned appearance. She didn't look overweight, and if she had never stepped on a bathroom scale, she would never have thought she had a weight problem.

The term "overweight" is obsolete. We realize now that fat can be hidden inside the body in such a way that some people can carry a lot of excess fat without seeming overweight at all. And other people, who fight to lose weight all their lives, never realize that they're *supposed* to weigh a lot because they have big bones and big muscles.

8

How to Calculate Your Correct Weight

Now comes the fun part. Having calculated how much lean you have, you can calculate how much you should weigh. Figuring your correct weight from those old-fashioned height/weight charts is useless, because height alone doesn't account for the fact that naturally heavy-boned, heavily muscled people can weigh proportionately more. The ONLY WAY to predict your correct weight is to add the proper amount of fat to your lean body mass. For men, we divide pounds of lean body mass by .85, which is the arithmetic way to add 15 percent. For women, we divide lean by .78, which is the same as adding 22 percent.

Men: pounds of lean ÷ .85 = correct weight to be 15% fat
Women: pounds of lean ÷ .78 = correct weight to be 22% fat

Example: When Ann and Jack were body fat tested, Ann's fat was 25 percent and Jack's was 18 percent, both 3 percent higher than what Covert recommends. How much should they weigh in order to be a healthy 22 percent (for her) and a healthy 15 percent fat (for him)?

As the chart on page 43 shows, Ann and Jack have nearly the same amount of fat, but Jack has 33 more pounds of lean. To be a healthy 22 percent fat, Ann needs to lose 5 pounds, while Jack, to be a healthy 15 percent fat, needs to lose 6 pounds.

	Ann	Jack
Total weight	130 lbs.	160 lbs.
% fat	25%	18%
Fat	32 lbs.	29 lbs.
	$(130 \times .25 = 32)$	$(160 \times .18 = 29)$
Lean	98 lbs.	131 lbs.
	$(130 - 32 = 98)$	$(160 - 29 = 131)$
Ideal weight	125 lbs. (to be 22% fat)	154 lbs. (to be 15% fat)
	$(98 \div .78 = 125)$	$(131 \div .85 = 154)$

When people find out how much they should weigh based on their current pounds of lean, they react in one of three ways. About a third say, "Yeah, that's about what I should weigh." They have a realistic idea of what their correct weight should be because they've *been* at that weight before and felt fit and healthy. Most of these people have done sports in the past, which gave them a realistic feel for their correct weight.

Another third are quite surprised that their correct weight is higher than they think it should be. They're the "heavy lean" guys or gals I mentioned earlier—people who think they're overweight but who have bigger bones and muscles than average. Yes, they may indeed be overweight, but not as much as they thought. I have a friend, Paul, who fits this category. He's a big man, six foot two, weighing 220 pounds. Right now he tests at 20 percent fat, which means he has 44 pounds of fat and 176 pounds of lean. To be a healthy 15 percent fat, Paul needs to weigh 207 pounds (176 ÷ .85). But Paul thinks 207 pounds would be much too heavy. Paul was a wrestler in high school and remembers his "fightin'" weight as 185 pounds. (Most male wrestlers are between 5 and 10

HE'S HOT, SHE'S COLD

Guys, how often does this happen? You and your wife get into the car on a chilly night, and the first thing she does is turn on the heater. Or she piles on blankets at night while you're sweating under a sheet. How come she's always cold while you're hot? If women are fatter than men, shouldn't that fat insulate them and keep them warmer?

Yes, women do have more skin fat than men, but it acts as a sort of reverse insulator, so that the heat they produce deep inside doesn't reach the skin surface as quickly. So women "feel" cold easily. They are not colder in the body core than men. In the examples above, it's the superficial skin temperature that makes women feel cold, not their core temperature.

In frigid survival situations, women often fare better than men. Their sensation of cold comes on more quickly, but their core is better insulated. Men in frigid conditions produce more heat (burn more calories) because they have more lean mass, but they lose all that heat quickly through their thinner layer of fat.

All this discussion of body heat just emphasizes that metabolism and calories burned depend mostly on muscle. No diet is ever going to increase the quantity or quality of muscle.

---

percent fat.) If Paul got back to his high school weight (given his present amount of lean) he would be 5 percent fat! At the age of fifty-three, Paul has set an unrealistic goal for himself, one that would be extremely difficult to attain. Instead of trying to lose 35 pounds in order to reach his teenage 5 percent fat level, he should lose only 13 pounds.

Finally, about a third of the people tested aren't at all pleased when they find out how much they should weigh. That's because their correct weight is much *lower* than what they think it should be. These are the "skinny fatsos" who have lost muscle over the years. Their present frames can't afford to carry as much weight as they did in the past. While women fall into this group more often than men, I'll never forget one man who was skinny but fat. Bruce was six feet tall and weighed 150 pounds. He was thin to the point of looking gaunt. He had never done anything athletic in his life and ate huge amounts of food in an attempt to gain weight. He didn't look fat, but his underexercised muscles were loaded with the stuff. Bruce tested at 24 percent fat, and we shocked everyone in the clinic when we told him that his correct weight should be 134 pounds! You can imagine his reaction. "Why, if I weighed that little I'd look sick!" he complained. "You're right!" I answered, "but right now you are sick, because you have too much fat compared to your lean." Of course, I don't *really* want people like Bruce to lose weight. I want them to do something to regain the muscle they've lost and get rid of the excess fat.

9 What Is the Cure for All This Fat?

Plant firmly in your head the fact that the problem is not excess fat; fat is only the outer symptom. The real problem is the lack of fat-burning muscle underneath the fat. As muscle gives way to fat, not only does muscle decrease, thereby lessening the need for calories, but also the chemistry of the remaining muscle changes in such a way as to require fewer calories.

Dieting may decrease fat, but it cannot increase the amount of muscle or reverse the badly altered chemistry of the muscles. Additionally, dieting does nothing to improve body shape. If a person was fat and pear-shaped before a diet, he'll be skinny and pear-shaped afterward.

Dieting attacks subcutaneous fat first; intramuscular fat is lost only under the most severe prison-camp conditions. Even if you were willing to undergo such rigor, the results would be disappointing, because you wouldn't have done anything to keep from getting fat all over again. Furthermore, your situation might actually be worse; radical dieting, unbalanced dieting, shots, and fasting have been shown to *decrease* muscle mass while a person loses fat.

We have developed such a mania for losing weight that we overlook what the lost weight consists of. Suppose I were to call you on the telephone with the exciting news that the local supermarket was selling twelve pounds for only $1.29!

Your reaction would be, "Twelve pounds of what?" Well, that's what I ask when someone tells me of a terrific diet that guarantees you will lose twelve pounds in no time at all—twelve pounds of what? Unfortunately, while losing fat, you may also lose muscle, which decreases the need for calories and makes the problem worse.

All of us can think of someone we know who has gone on a diet only to end up looking gaunt and haggard. We admonish the person that she really would look better with a little more fat. But it isn't the loss of fat that gives her a wasted appearance, it's the loss of muscle! No, dieting isn't the cure for excess fat.

While many people diet to get rid of fat, a handful of people do just the opposite. They look skinny, so they *overeat* to gain weight. But when one does this, the added weight is only *fat*. The waistline disappears, the arms get flabby, the thighs and buttocks fatten up, and a double chin may even develop. Overeating to gain weight will add fat and put it in places where you need it the least.

ONE MORE BREAK!

Okay, we're just about ready to home in on my exercise program, so this will be the last of your "unsupervised" breaks. After this you'll be designing a program that's just right for you. So now go out for another ten-minute walk. Nothing silly this time — we don't want the neighbors calling the loony bin. As you walk, don't think about all this stuff you've been reading. If your body fat test came out too high, don't worry about it. I'm going to show you how to get rid of your fat. Just think about how good the fresh air smells, how sweetly the birds are singing, how warm the sun feels. And if you live in Oregon, as I do, well, have fun splashing in the puddles.

Compare these overeaters and un-
dereaters to the many people who
have exercised their bodies to low fat
levels. They are full-bodied, healthy in-

> The ultimate cure for fat is exercise!

dividuals who lead active lives without being constantly con-
cerned about the number of calories they eat.

Exercise increases muscle, tones it, alters its chemistry,
and increases the metabolic rate. All of these effects mean
that you burn more calories even when you're asleep.

10 What Kind of Exercise Is Best?

If you want to get fit and lose fat, find a twelve-year-old kid. Whatever he does — you do! If he runs around the block, you run around the block. If he climbs a tree, you climb a tree. Kids zoom here and there, getting fit while tearing up the house. They never stop to say, "Oh! I must do my jogging now!" or "I should go to my aerobics class now." If we all did what most young kids do, we wouldn't need to read books like this.

Okay, okay, I know that most of us don't have the time to play like kids. We have work, we have family obligations. We need the kind of exercise that pays big fat-loss dividends with minimum time invested. We need to find exercise that gives us the most for our money, so to speak. I'm going to describe that kind of exercise, but as I do, keep in mind that the BEST exercise is the one that makes you feel like a kid again — because then you will smile, be happy, and do lots of it.

The most *efficient* exercise to get rid of fat, which is the most efficient way to change your metabolism so you won't get fat anymore, is gentle nonstop exercise. More specifically, you need to do exercise that gets you breathing deeply but does not leave you out of breath; that is continuous and uninterrupted; and that uses the big muscles of the thighs and buttocks. Right away you should be able to name several examples, such as walking, jogging, bicycling, and cross-country skiing.

Exercises like these, which are gentle and nonstop, train muscles to burn fat and, more important, they change your metabolism so you won't get fat anymore. Why wouldn't hard, intense exercises have the same effect? The answer has to do with breathing. When you exercise to the point of breathing deeply but not getting out of breath, your muscles burn fat. When you exercise so hard that you get out of breath, your muscles stop burning fat.

Pay attention now; this is the big point of this chapter, and perhaps the biggest point of the whole book:

Muscles burn fat ONLY ONLY ONLY in the presence of oxygen. When you get out of breath, fat-burning shuts down.

Muscles burn two kinds of fuel—fat and sugar (glucose). They prefer to burn fat because it lasts a long time and produces lots of energy, but fat can't be burned unless the muscles get oxygen.

When the muscles need quick energy, they switch to burning sugar. In contrast to fat, sugar/glucose can be burned *without* oxygen. When you run fast enough to get out of breath, your muscles are deprived of oxygen. It seems odd, doesn't it? Even though you are breathing hard, the oxygen supply to the muscles isn't sufficient for fat metabolism to continue. When there's not enough oxygen for fat-burning, sugar-burning takes over.

Scientists call the oxygen-dependent burning of fat "aerobic metabolism," and, based on that phenomenon, the term "aerobic exercise" was coined.

Aerobic Exercise (to the Layman)
Gets you breathing deeply but doesn't get you out of breath.
Is steady and nonstop.
Uses the big muscles of the thighs and buttocks.

Aerobic Exercise (to the Scientist)
Provides plenty of oxygen to the muscles, which
Promotes fat burning in the muscles, which
Makes you a better butter-burner!

The simple explanation I have offered so far needs a little expansion. In reality, muscles burn fat and sugar at the same time, but they *prefer* to burn fat during gentle activity, and they *prefer* to burn sugar/glucose during intense activity. In other words, hard, out-of-breath exercise burns some fat, but it's not the *most efficient way* to burn fat.

There's another aspect of aerobic exercise that is much more important than how much fat it burns while you're doing it.

Enzymes are specialized proteins found in muscle tissue. Some enzymes are specifically designed to burn fat, while others burn sugar. When you exercise gently, the fat-burning enzymes do most of the work. When you exercise hard and get out of breath, the sugar-burning enzymes take over. They're sort of like labor unions. The fat-burning-enzyme union says, "Sure, we'll burn fat as long as she gives us enough oxygen. But no oxygen—no work!" And they go on strike.

The enzymes in the fat-burning union are basically lazy. Not only do they go on strike if you exercise too hard, they also lay off workers when you don't exercise at all. If you go for months without exercising, the number of fat-burning enzymes diminishes. This means that what used to

> Aerobic exercise stimulates the growth of fat-burning enzymes, so you tend to burn more fat even when you're sitting around doing nothing. In other words, a fit person burns more fat — while he or she is resting — than a fat person does.

be gentle, not-out-of-breath exercise may now be too intense for you; you get out of breath more easily than you used to. It also means that you have lost much of your fat-burning potential.

If you have lost your fat-burning capabilities because you haven't exercised for a long time, you need to find a way to get the fat-burning-enzyme union to hire more workers (create new enzymes). To do that you have to make them work, which to them is aerobic exercise. You need to do lots of gentle exercise that doesn't get you out of breath. As long as you supply them with enough oxygen, the fat-burning enzymes will work. But they won't like it! Remember, they're basically lazy. They complain, "She keeps jogging every day! But she doesn't go so fast that we can let the sugar-burning enzymes take over. We need more workers!" And so, to make the work easier, your muscles "hire on" new fat-burning enzymes. As these enzymes increase, you find that you can exercise a little harder before you get out of breath.

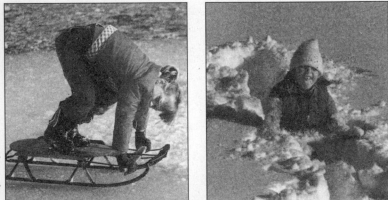

Sally Bailey

Christina Bailey, 1982
If you want to get fit fast, find a twelve-year-old kid. Whatever he she does, you do!

When you can exercise harder without getting out of breath, then you're burning MORE fat. And, more important, you're making more fat-burning enzymes, which means that you are slowly changing your body into a fat-burning machine. You are becoming a better butter-burner!

I recommend the activities below. They are *always* aerobic in nature; it's easy to do them right and hard to do them wrong. You may have a unique personal aerobic exercise — maybe you enjoy high-speed running on the moon — but the ones I recommend here are tried and familiar friends, and they don't require a spaceship.

Aerobic Exercises

Running/jogging

Hiking

Cross-country skiing

Water aerobics

Mountain biking

Rowing

Race walking

Walking

Swimming

Jumping rope

Bicycling

Aerobics classes

Machines

Treadmill

Cross-country ski machine

Aerobic rider

Stationary bicycle

Stair climber

Rowing machine

Step/ladder climber

Mini-trampoline

Elliptical machine

Nonaerobic Exercises

The activities listed on the next page are not generally considered aerobic, although some people modify them to derive aerobic benefits. Very fit people, for example, make good use of stop-and-go sports such as basketball and racquetball to build and maintain fitness. In contrast, low-key activities such as golf yield little aerobic benefit unless you're elderly or unfit or both. For now, stick with the list of aerobic exercises on page 53.

Racquetball/squash	Soccer
Downhill skiing	Horseback riding
Baseball	In-line skating
Field/ice hockey	Water skiing
Motorcycle riding	Football
Tennis	Ice skating
Windsurfing	Golf
Volleyball	Basketball
Dancing	Gymnastics

11 Measuring Exercise by Heart Rate

Aerobic exercise needs to be:

- Gentle enough so that the muscles burn fat rather than sugar.
- Hard enough to stimulate the growth of new fat-burning enzymes.

In other words, for exercise to be aerobic, it mustn't be too slow and it mustn't be too fast. But how slow is too slow and how fast is too fast? By determining that, you can get the most from your exercise by staying between the two extremes.

The aerobic zone is quite broad. The obvious question is, "How do I know if I'm exercising in the zone?" Well, your heart beats faster and faster the harder you exercise, so taking your pulse (heart rate) during exercise works quite well. To do this accurately, however, you have to know how fast your heart beats at maximum. Everyone's maximum is different. It may be that when you are exercising at full bore, your heart beats 200 times a minute, but my heart won't go faster than 135 beats a minute. So exercising at 120 beats per minute would feel very different for each of us. You can find books and lecturers advising that exercise must be at a specific heart rate, as if we were all the same. What foolishness!

Ideally, you should find out your own maximum heart

rate. One way to do this is by taking an expensive treadmill test, complete with attending physicians and resuscitating paddles. Once you have established your maximum heart rate, exercising between 65 and 80 percent of that number will put you in the aerobic zone, which means you will be burning fat AND stimulating the growth of new fat-burning enzymes.

But there is a simpler method, using the following formula:

220 minus your age = maximum heart rate

In other words, age and heart rate are related. Using this formula, you first determine your maximum heart rate, then multiply that number by 65 percent and 80 percent to get the range of how fast your heart should beat during aerobic exercise.

maximum heart rate × .65 = low end of aerobic zone

maximum heart rate × .80 = high end of aerobic zone

Ideal Exercise Heart Rate = 65–80% of maximum

Practically every gym in America has a listing of age-related exercise heart rates like the one shown on the next page.

To get the biggest payoff from your exercise (which means lots of fat-burning and an increase in enzymes), you should work hard enough to make your heart beat at least at 65 percent but at no more than 80 percent of the maximum for your age. According to the chart, if you are forty, your maximum heart rate would be 180, and you should exercise hard enough to get your heart beating in the range between 117 and 144 beats per minute.

Let's consider three forty-year-old men. The first is terribly out of shape, which means he has a lot of intramuscular fat as well as some obvious subcutaneous fat bulging under

Recommended Heart Rate During Aerobic Exercise*

Age	Maximum heart rate	65–80% of maximum	If you have a history of heart disease, DO NOT EXCEED 65% of maximum
20	200	130–160	130
25	195	127–156	127
30	190	124–152	124
35	185	120–148	120
40	180	117–144	117
45	175	114–140	114
50	170	111–136	111
55	165	107–132	107
60	160	104 128	104
65+	150	98–120	98

*Not everyone fits this chart! Please read this chapter before you use it!

his skin. He might easily drive his pulse to 144 just by walking briskly. The second man, in better shape, might have to jog to get 144 beats per minute. And the third man, lean and athletic, might have to run at quite a fast pace to reach the same heart rate. You may think that the third man is getting the most exercise, while the first man is being lazy. But in fact they are all exercising equally, getting the same heart, lung, and muscular benefits.

For years the fat man who has tried to jog with his trim friend has felt he must jog at the same speed to get the same exercise. Now he can see that he should walk, jog, or run at whatever speed gives him the correct heart rate.

TIPS ON DOING HEART-RATE-MONITORED EXERCISE

Let me again caution you: heart-rate-monitored exercise may not be right for you. If you have to exercise very hard to reach the recommended heart rate, *don't use this method!* If you feel as if you're hardly exercising at all when you reach the recommended heart rate, *don't use this method*. If you have a pacemaker or are using heart-rate-regulating drugs, *don't use this method*.

- First, learn how to take your resting pulse. If you become familiar with finding your pulse when you're sitting quietly, it will be that much easier to find when you're exercising and your heart is beating more vigorously.

- You can find your pulse by placing your fingertips gently on the thumb side of your wrist. If it's difficult to find the pulse there, as is often the case in women and older people, try one side of your neck. (Don't press both sides at once.) Your fingers will pick up the pulse. Don't use your thumb. It has its own pulse, and you might get a double count.

- Once you have found the pulse, count it for exactly 6 seconds. Multiply the number of beats you counted by 10. Most people get a count of 60, 70, 80, or 90. Take your pulse again, and this time be careful to note whether you were between numbers at the end of 6 seconds. With practice you should be able to count half beats or even quarter beats. For example, suppose you count your pulse as "One, two, three, four, five, six, and one-half." That's a pulse of 65.

continued

Athletic husbands are often guilty of pushing their wives into too-strenuous exercise. The man coerces his wife into going out for "just a little jog together." He runs slower for her and she runs faster for him. One is underexercised, the other

- This is your resting pulse. You should take your pulse several times during the day to get your average resting pulse. Most women average 80 beats per minute, and most men about 72 beats a minute. There's that word "average" again. It may be average to have a resting pulse of either 72 or 80, but it would be healthier and normal to have a much lower resting pulse. As you become more fit, your resting pulse rate will drop.

- Now you're ready to take your pulse during exercise. And now you'll see why I've had you practice taking 6-second pulses instead of the usual 15-second count. During exercise, you'll have to stop momentarily to take your pulse (unless you're on a stationary bicycle). As you relax, your heart starts to relax also, and your heart rate quickly slows down. If you count for the usual 15 seconds, the count will be completely false because your heart will be beating faster at the beginning of the count than at the end.

- To be aerobic, your exercise should be vigorous enough to get your pulse above 65 percent but below 80 percent of the maximum rate for your age. If your pulse is slower or faster than this range, increase or decrease your exertion accordingly.

- At first you'll want to check your exercise pulse several times during your workout to become familiar with how to do it and with how your heart rate relates to your overall breathing and exertion. Once you know how hard you should exercise to reach your training zone, you need only check your pulse at the end of your workout.

is overexercised, and it is inefficient exercise for both of them. Men and women should think twice about exercising together because of the difference in their muscle mass. Even if a man and a woman are carrying approximately the same amount of fat, he has a much bigger "engine" to carry it.

Heart-rate-monitored exercise is useful, but there's a problem with the 220-minus-age formula; it fits only about 60 percent of the population. Approximately 15 percent of us have hearts that beat considerably slower than the predicted maximum and another 15 percent have hearts that beat much faster. This doesn't mean there's anything wrong with these hearts or that they are abnormal. It just means they aren't *average*.

> Often people ask me if it's okay to use a heart-rate monitor. I say, sure! They're fun and easy to use, but you still want to be competent at taking your pulse. You won't always remember your heart-rate monitor, but your fingers are with you all the time.

Let's say your heart beats faster than average during exercise. If you're thirty years old, you would expect your heart to beat 220 minus 30, or 190, beats a minute when you exercise at maximum. But yours beats at 210. It's as if you had a hummingbird heart: it's built very well, but it's made to function at a high RPM. When you exercise, your heart goes much faster than all the charts say it should, and your aerobics instructor is afraid you're going to die any minute. You're not going to die—you just have a heart that beats very fast and is therefore off the chart. If you were to exercise at the heart rate recommended for your age, you would be exercising too slowly to derive aerobic benefits.

Similarly, the 15 percent of the population whose hearts beat slower than average at maximum would be exercising much too hard to derive aerobic benefits if they used the formula and/or the charts. I fall into this category. My maximum heart rate according to the formula should be around 150–155 beats per minute, but try as hard as I can, it never exceeds 135. If I were to exercise at 80 percent of the formula-predicted maximum heart rate, I'd be exercising at practically maximum exertion.

Finally, 10 percent of the population (I'm only guessing at this number) is taking medication that affects heart rate. These people's heart rates may fit the formula, but the medication artificially depresses their heart rate during exercise. Pulse monitoring as a measure of exercise intensity is not reliable for this group either.

After all these caveats, you may wonder why I even bother to talk about heart-rate-monitored exercise. There must be a better way. There is! It's called "exercise using common sense," and I'll teach you how to do it in the next chapter. But heart-rate-monitored exercise has been used for years and years, and it DOES have value in that it teaches you a sort of body awareness. If you couple it with my "common-sense" approach, you will have an extremely accurate method of determining *your personally correct* aerobic level of exercise.

12 Exercise Using Common Sense

Aerobic Exercise Measured by the Talk Test

A simple way to find your correct level of exercise is to do the "talk test." Say you are jogging with a friend. Is he able to talk while you are not? Each of you should be able to talk a little bit, but neither of you should be able to sing an aria. For fun, try singing, "Row, Row, Row Your Boat." If you can't get beyond the second "Row" without gasping for breath, you're exercising too hard. On the other hand, if you get past "gently down the stream" before you need to take a breath, you should speed up.

When I'm coaching beginners, I jog along beside them asking questions. "What's your name? Where are you from? What did you have for dinner last night?" I want to hear three- and four-word responses, not lengthy dissertations or one-word gasps. Try it yourself. When you're walking, jogging, bicycling, or cross-country skiing, pretend Covert Bailey is with you asking all sorts of questions. Any time you find you can't talk in short three- and four-word phrases because you are either exercising so hard you're out of breath or so gently you're becoming a chatterbox, slow down or speed up as necessary.

If you exercise according to your breathing, you are just using common sense. As you exercise, think to yourself, "Am I doing something that makes my fat-burning enzymes burn fat? Or are they turning the job over to the sugar-burning enzymes because I'm out of breath and there's no oxygen in my muscles?" If you are able to talk haltingly while breathing deeply but comfortably, you are almost certainly exercising aerobically with your heart beating between 65 and 80 percent of its maximum. But I mean your *true* maximum heart rate that a laboratory treadmill test would determine—not the hypothetical maximum derived from the formula (220 − age = maximum).

Now! Let's put breathing and heart rate together. Once you have found a comfortable exercise intensity according to your breathing, take your pulse. For 60 percent of you, the pulse you get will be between 65 and 80 percent of the formula 220 minus your age (maximum heart rate). For the other 40 percent, your heart rate will be higher or lower than the one predicted by the formula. If you're one of these people, don't speed up or slow down to adjust your heart rate. Instead, stick with the pace that keeps you breathing deeply but not gasping. In other words, trust your breathing (the talk test) more than your heart rate. If we could test you on a treadmill for your true maximum heart rate, we would probably find that even though your exercise heart rate is slower or faster than what the formula says it should be, it is the correct

---

Once, while lecturing to a group of physicians, I made the following statement to see if they were listening: "Fat people should exercise as hard as they possibly can ..." (long pause)

I could see some of the doctors having heart attacks just thinking about all the fat people who were going to have heart attacks if they followed my advice.

Before the doctors could start throwing things at me, I added, "Fat people should exercise as hard as they can ... *WITHOUT ever getting out of breath.*"

> Trust your breathing (the talk test) more than your heart rate.

rate FOR YOU. The value of using the breathing method to determine exercise heart rate is that it's YOUR aerobic heart rate, not a hypothetical one derived from a generic formula.

There are several advantages to monitoring your heart rate and your breathing during exercise. Suppose you're exercising at your regular speed but breathing harder than you usually do. When you take your pulse, it will probably be higher than usual. Maybe you're tired or your body is trying to fight off a virus. Whatever the reason, your body is telling you that your usual exercise level is too intense for that particular day. You should slow down until your heart is beating at its usual exercise pace.

You can also monitor your breathing/heart rate to make adjustments for exercising at higher altitudes. You may be tempted to exercise at your usual speed when you're in the mountains, but if you check your breathing and heart rate, you'll realize you should slow down.

Macho types don't think they need to bother with the talk test. They have the notion that exercise is useless unless it induces labored breathing. When I try the talk test on one of these die-hards, he assures me that he's exercising aerobically. "Oh, I'm not out of breath *(gasp, gasp)* I'm just *(wheeze, gasp, cough)* breathing deeply *(wheeze, choke, gasp)* to get oxygen to my muscles *(cough, gasp, wheeze)* so they'll burn lots of fat!!! *(sputter, sputter, wheeze)*." Buddy, your fat-burning enzymes went on strike long ago. You are burning zero fat!

13 Covert Bailey's Fitness Test

I'm going to describe a home fitness test that costs nothing, is self-administered, and doesn't hurt. In a sense, "my" test isn't mine at all, because joggers already use it. When people who jog for fitness discuss their daily run, it is common to hear them use the word "pace." They are referring to the average number of minutes it takes them to jog a mile.

Pace, or minutes per mile, does not imply maximum. Asking a jogger her pace is not at all the same as asking, "How fast can you run a mile?" Quite the opposite. It means "How fast can you run a mile without discomfort *and do the same tomorrow and again the next day?*" Among those who jog almost every day, the routine number of minutes per mile becomes just that — routine. Their pace is a consistently reliable number, and it is an excellent indicator of their fitness.

An Olympic runner can sprint a mile in four minutes, can race consecutive five-minute miles, and can run comfortably at a six-minute-per-mile aerobic pace. That runner would be wrong to claim he had a five-minute pace or a four-minute pace. Those are his racing and sprinting times; his steady aerobic pace is six minutes.

We can compare pace with driving speed. On the freeway with no traffic and no cops, do you tend to cruise at fifty-five or sixty? At what speed does the engine purr? I have a nice car and an ancient pickup. The car always seems to want to go sixty-five or more, but I have to make an effort to push the pickup to go even fifty-five. My old pickup isn't fit anymore, so its pace, or cruising speed, is a little slow.

Some may criticize the pace concept on the grounds that it depends too much on personal motivation and sensation, but for people who jog, pace is incredibly accurate. It's exactly the comfort zone of the individual, and no formula or laboratory can do better. Obviously, if you are not a regular runner and you try to determine your pace in a single day, you've missed the point.

I want *everyone* to determine his or her own pace. It's not something just for jocks. Young, old, fit, not-so-fit — everyone should know his pace. It should be something you check as routinely as you do your weight. Imagine what a boon it would be to your doctor to know your pace.

When you go to your physician for a checkup, he does all kinds of tests to get an assessment of your overall health. But the most important thing he wants is — to SEE you. He's not satisfied just with urinalysis, blood analysis, and all the other tests. He wants to look at you, because a visual assessment can often better describe a patient than a battery of tests. Your doctor might write only a few words on your chart. "The patient appeared *frail*." Or *robust*, or *vital*. It would take a paragraph to define each of those words, because each has a world of meaning.

Pace, or cruising speed, is like that; it tells a great deal about a person. Even if I have never met you, if you tell me on the telephone that your pace is eight, nine, or ten minutes a mile, I have an instant visual image of you. I know you are not fat, you are vital, and your metabolism allows you to eat almost anything you want. If you tell me that your pace is twenty or twenty-five minutes a mile, I would suspect that you are fat, old, or, perhaps, ill.

> Pace, or cruising speed, is an excellent measure of one's health.

Someday, if this book is convincing enough, pace, or cruising speed, will be a measure used by everybody, not just the very fit. Our doctors will add it to their list of examination words. Someday, if my dreams come true, I will be looking at someone's medical records and there will be "The patient's pace is 14 minutes a mile." The pace number had to come from the patient to the doctor, not the other way around. And I'll breathe a sigh of relief, knowing that both the doctor and the patient realize that pace is an excellent measure of health.

Once each of us becomes familiar with the pace concept and observant of fluctuations in our own pace, we will be able to talk about health in a whole new way. People will say things like this:

"My pace is usually a ten-minute mile, but I had a wicked cold last month and I'm down to eleven."

"I plateaued at twelve minutes a mile for nearly a year. Couldn't seem to improve until I switched to a different exercise, then I improved to ten!"

"I can't believe it! I've gone from sixteen to fifteen minutes a mile in two weeks just by eating less fat."

How to Determine Your Pace

It will take you at least five days to do my fitness test. First, find a level, flat mile. A high school or college track is best because it is one-quarter mile around, so you can measure the distance quite precisely. If you can't find a track nearby, measure one mile on a level road with your car. Then walk/jog/run each day for five days and keep a record of how long it takes you to cover the mile. If you're young and fit, do the test five days in a row. If you're older and/or out of condition, do it every other day until you have five days' worth.

The key to this test is that it must be done at a comfortable aerobic pace. If you've never measured your pace before, I suggest that you do it for seven days, because the first two days won't be accurate. People who aren't used to determining pace tend to push themselves a little more than they normally would for the first couple of days.

After five days, average the time you spent exercising. For example:

Minutes to Cover 1 Mile

Sunday	Monday	Tuesday	Thursday	Friday
15	15½	14½	15	15

Total time (over 5 days) = 75 minutes

75 ÷ 5 = pace of 15 minutes a mile

Remember, your goal is not to try to run harder each day but rather to establish a comfortable aerobic pace. By the end of a week, you should have a good idea of your pace.

> Your pace is not how fast you can run a mile. It's the speed at which you walk, jog, or run mile after mile after mile.

Pace becomes more accurate when you are able to go farther than one mile. Runners who can cover three or four miles find it easy to calculate their pace accurately. If one mile is too far for you, your pace will be less accurate. I urge you — do the test anyway! Suppose you can walk only a half mile. You can figure your minutes-per-mile pace by doubling the time it takes you to walk the half mile.

You may be reluctant to do this, saying, "I already know I'm out of shape. I don't need to take a test to prove it." In spite of its inaccuracy with very unfit people, pace is quite useful in monitoring progress. And the more out of shape a person is, the more pronounced his or her progress will be.

Superfit athletes have to work extremely hard to improve their pace. To advance from a six-minute pace to a five-and-a-half-minute pace requires months and months of hard training. At the opposite end of the scale, however, unfit people get huge leaps in performance in a short time. If your current pace is a thirty-minute mile, you will quickly drop to a twenty-five-minute mile after just a week or so of gentle exercise. Instead of being discouraged because your pace is slow, look at the positive side. While Mr. Super Athlete busts his gut to shave a few *seconds* off his pace, you can knock two or three *minutes* off your pace in no time at all!

Out-of-condition people often don't realize how much they are improving when they start an exercise program. After their initial excitement, they quickly get discouraged because it seems as if they aren't making progress. They see

How Fit Are You?

Your aerobic pace*	Fitness level		Covert's comments
	−45 years	45 years+	
6 minutes	Olympic caliber, very high		People in this section are exceptionally fit, but they have to exercise long and hard to stay that way. It's great if you can do it, but it's probably not a realistic goal for most busy working people.
7–8 minutes	High	Very high	If your aerobic pace is eight minutes or less, you can subtract 3% from your body fat percentage (calculated in Chapter 5).
9–10 minutes	Above average	High	This is what I call the good-health section. People under age 45 should be able to run, jog, or walk a mile in 9–13 minutes; people over 45 should be able to do it in 9–17 minutes.
11–13 minutes	Average	Above average	
14–17 minutes	Below average	Average	
18–20 minutes	Poor	Below average	If you fall into this section, take heart. You can make dramatic improvements with only moderate effort. No excuses! Don't say you can't because you're too fat or too old or too this or too that.
21 minutes or longer	Very poor	Poor	Close this book right now, get up out of your chair, go outside, and start walking — NOW!

*Remember! Aerobic pace is how fast you run, jog, or walk consecutive miles at a comfortable pace that doesn't get you out of breath.

their fit friends running for miles, while all they can do is take short walks. If they walk in one direction one day and another direction the next, they never get a feel for their distance or speed. By keeping track of their pace, they'll see that enormous changes are occurring.

Again, I urge you to determine your pace, even if you're fat and out of shape. Keep track of it. Recheck it often. I guarantee that if you exercise according to the methods I've described in this book, you will be surprised at how quickly your pace improves.

Here's How to Get Started
- Pick two aerobic exercises.
- Exercise four or five days a week (two days on, one day off, and so on).
- Exercise for at least twenty minutes each session.
- Instead of doing the same aerobic exercise each time, switch back and forth between your two selections.
- This is your "basic fitness program." Beginners, continue with this program for four to six weeks BEFORE you add different or additional exercises.

Beginners, please! Don't be tempted to jump ahead. Your body needs time to adjust to the exercises. It needs time to grow those fat-burning enzymes we talked about. It needs rest and recuperation days. If you follow my recommendations you will find that starting *and continuing with* an exercise program is easy and lots of fun! These beginning recommendations will be modified in later chapters.

15 Choosing Your Aerobic Exercise

Keep in mind as you read the following descriptions that whole-body exercises are the ones that use lots of muscle, ones that not only get your big leg and buttocks muscles moving but that incorporate your arms and upper body as well. Weight-bearing exercises are the ones in which you're on your feet moving your weight from one place to another. While all aerobic exercises get you fit and induce the growth of fat-burning enzymes, the whole-body and weight-bearing exercises usually give quicker results.

Types of Aerobic Exercise

Aerobics Classes

I really like aerobics classes because people of varying degrees of fitness can exercise together, each at his or her own pace. The variety of classes is endless — step, low/high impact, dance, slide, funk—but they all have one thing in common: they're fun! The hour you spend in an aerobics class seems to fly by. How many other kinds of aerobic exercise would you routinely do for an hour? The "stick-to-it" rate is higher with aerobics classes than with any other exercise.

A well-constructed aerobics class includes stretching, aerobics, cross training, high-intensity work, and modified weight training. You burn up lots of fat in the weight-bearing, whole-body portion of the class, then work your muscles during the floor exercises. And the bonus you get with aerobics classes that you don't always get with other forms of exercise is better coordination and proprioception. (There's more on these topics later in this chapter.)

You say you can't get to a class? There are lots of aerobics videotapes available.

Running/Jogging/Racewalking

These exercises yield both whole-body and weight-bearing benefits, making them excellent for rapid fat loss. BUT! If you're very heavy or very unfit, they're too strenuous (and potentially dangerous). Wait until you're lighter and fitter before trying these.

If you do jog or run, you can minimize your risk of injury by varying the length of your stride, your speed, and your foot strike. Vary your style by skipping or running sideways or backward. Run on softer surfaces, such as wood-chip trails, composition, or rubberized asphalt.

Walking

I deliberately separated walking from running/jogging because they are *not* the same. Although both forms of exercise are weight-bearing, walking tends to be a slow fat-burner. It's good for beginners and older people, but the young and/or fit have to wear a backpack or find hilly routes to get aerobic benefits from walking.

Bicycling

Bicycling is neither weight-bearing nor a whole-body exercise. It will get you fit, but you'll have to bike for long periods to burn significant amounts of fat. That changes if you're an enthusiast of mountain biking, for you have to use practically every muscle in your body to zig and zag through the woods, jump over rocks, and grind up hills.

Cross-Country Skiing

The king of aerobic exercises! Cross-country skiing is the fastest fat-burner and is more strenuous than running, yet the risk of injury is low because the movements are gliding rather than pounding. You'll be surprised how hard you work, even though your pace is usually slower than your jogging/running pace. But, of course, the big drawback is that it's seasonal.

Rowing

This non-weight-bearing exercise is one of the best whole-body exercises. Like cross-country skiing, it exercises most of the large muscle groups without stress on joints and has the added benefit of developing the muscles of the upper torso. It's one of the few aerobic exercises that can be performed with one leg if you have an injury to the other.

Swimming and Water Aerobics

Swimming is great for increasing your fitness but poor for losing fat, because in water the body wants to keep its fat. (If you don't believe me, ask a seal!) If swimming is one of your aerobic exercises, be sure to combine it with a weight-bearing and/or whole-body exercise *on land*. Despite this drawback, I think swimming is a good way for fat people who are unused to exercise to start their program. They can learn body coordination and gain fitness without feeling clumsy or risking injury to already overburdened joints. Once they've built up a certain amount of coordination and fitness, they can venture on to exercises that burn more fat.

Swimming has other drawbacks. Beginners get out of breath easily, so it requires a lot of practice before you're good enough to get an aerobic workout. It's also hard to make swimming a nonstop exercise when you're in a pool full of people. The novice should try water aerobics classes as an alternative. They're much more fun than swimming laps.

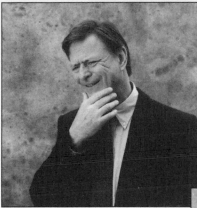

Imagine a fox and a seal having a conversation. The seal says, "I don't get it. How come I have all this fat? I *know* I'm fit. Last weekend I swam all the way to the Aleutian Islands just to see a girlfriend!"

"Furthermore, my doctor checked my arteries and said I'd never have a heart attack. I should be as skinny as you, Mr. Fox."

So the fox says, "Let's have a race to see who's fitter."

They both jump into the water, and the fox sinks like a rock.

The seal says, "Oh! I get it! I have a *life preserver!*"

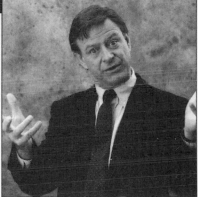

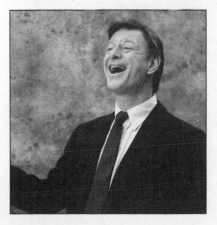

There's a center in the brain for fat control. If you run and run and run, that center says, "Dump everything! Get rid of the fat! Burn it off!" But if you swim all the time, the center says, *"Keep the life preserver!"*

Exercising against the water's resistance strengthens muscles without bumping and jarring. The buoyancy of the water keeps you from making fast, jerky, potentially injury-inducing motions. Since most of the workout is in the shallow end of the pool, even nonswimmers can join in. Water aerobics is great for everybody, but it has special advantages for older, fat, pregnant, or arthritic people.

Jumping Rope

Jumping rope is definitely weight-bearing — to the point of being very traumatic. Whole-body? Not really. It's a hard exercise to master and, unfortunately, once you get good at it you don't burn as much fat because your movements become so smooth and efficient you use less and less muscle. I don't make it one of my usual exercises, but I do like to carry a jump rope when I travel, to use in my hotel room when I don't want to run on unfamiliar streets.

The Machines

The difference between using a stationary bicycle and bicycling outdoors is subtle. When you ride a bicycle you do more than simply pedal. Your entire body is needed for balance, for last-second swerves, and for corrections to miss objects in your path. When your left leg pushes, your right leg counterbalances the motion, your arms steady the handlebars, your torso pushes forward. In effect, you train more muscles and more nerves than you do on a stationary bicycle.

This is also true when you run outside instead of using a treadmill. On a treadmill, your foot strikes the same way over and over again. Your stride is exactly the same. Some people even hold on to the front bar, thus getting no balance development at all. Contrast that with jogging outdoors. Your feet and ankles twist and turn in every direction, and your stride

---

COORDINATION

One of the advantages of an aerobics class is that it improves coordination. Aerobic machines such as treadmills, stair climbers, and stationary bikes, for which the movements are basically untrained and repetitive, do not require coordination. You just do what the machine guides you to do. Yes, you can get fit using these machines, and yes, you can lose fat. But you might end up as a fit, low-fat klutz!

Aerobic machines train the "gross" motor nerves — the large nerves responsible for ordinary locomotion. But they don't train the smaller, finer nerves that help you zig and zag down a ski slope. They don't train you for the balance you need to walk across a log over a stream while carrying a fifty-pound backpack. "But," you say, "I'm not a jock. I don't ski or backpack." Well, you still need coordination — just to square dance or play Frisbee with your kids!

Even if aerobics classes are not your favorite form of exercise, I'd like you to try them now and then. The erratic, back-and-forth, up-and-down movements are some of the best ways I know to develop coordination. By the way, aerobics classes aren't just dance-movement classes anymore. There are athletic-step classes, adventure-training classes, and even ski-conditioning classes.

---

is sometimes shortened, sometimes lengthened to adjust for obstacles. Your entire body constantly makes balance corrections with every step you take.

The point is that outdoor exercises requiring balance use more muscle while also helping to develop your coordination.

Does that mean you shouldn't use machines? Of course not! They're great if the weather is bad or if you're at home with young children. By changing the machine's speed and resistance, you can design exercise sessions that are just right

---

Exercise machines are good for rainy days, busy people, and the home-bound, but let's face it — nothing compares to the real thing. Stationary bicycling is exercise, but outdoor bicycling is sport. A treadmill is for exercise — a jog in the park is for fun. While both exercises will make you fit, outdoor activities give subtle benefits (such as balance and coordination) that you don't get with machines.

Most important, there's joy in outdoor sports. You incorporate them into your play. We happily throw our bikes on the roof of the car and take off for a day of cycling and picnicking with friends. But who would drag a stationary bicycle to a picnic??!!

---

for you instead of wasting time outdoors with downhills that are too easy or uphills that are too hard. And some of the newer machines include videos that give you the thrill of being in a bicycle race or a cross-country tour.

Treadmill

This is the perfect machine for both the beginning and the advanced exerciser. By varying the treadmill's speed and incline, you can do a fast, level jog one day and a steep, slower walk the next. Many people find that they can avoid the knee and back problems associated with jogging when they switch to a treadmill.

Aerobic Rider

This super-quiet machine is excellent for beginners, overweight people, and older people. It looks sort of like a stationary bicycle, but instead of pedaling, you push with your feet while pulling the handlebars. This action provides a whole-body, fat-burning effect by using every muscle in your body without producing soreness in any of them. In fact, it is one of the few machines you can use even if you're injured, because you can do it with one leg and two arms or one arm and two legs.

Stair Climber

This machine switches you back and forth between gentle aerobic exercise and more intense, muscle-building exercise. It doesn't provide true weight-bearing or whole-body exercise, but it is one of the better machines for burning off fat.

Elliptical Machine

This machine resembles a stair climber, but the motion is circular instead of up and down. It offers a wide variety of workouts, including some that are challenging to highly fit people and others that are fun for the not-so-fit. It is especially kind to joints, making it a good device to use when recovering from knee surgery.

Rowing Machine

This is a great machine for building upper-body muscle. For this reason, along with the strong leg movements it requires, it provides a whole-body fat-burning effect.

Cross-Country Ski Machine

This machine provides whole-body, weight-bearing exercise, which, of course, means lots of fat-burning. However, it requires skill and coordination to master it and takes up a lot of space.

Mini-Trampoline

This is a good piece of home equipment for people just starting out in an exercise program. For the already fit, it may not provide enough of a workout. You can vary your regular bouncing by running in place, jumping rope, or dancing to music on it. It's good for developing coordination and motor skills.

PROPRIOCEPTION

If you take a drunk-driving test, you have to put your hands out in front of you and touch your fingers together with your eyes closed. It's simple to do this when you're sober, but if you've been drinking too much the alcohol blurs the nerve signals in your arms and fingers so that they don't have a sense of where they are. There's a big word for this "sense of body position" — proprioception.

One of the neat things about very fit athletes is that they have a highly developed sense of body awareness. There is no way Michael Jordan could leap into the air, turn around three times, fake out all his opponents, and still do a perfect lay-up if the proprioceptors in his joints didn't tell him exactly where every part of his body was as he flew through the air.

People who keep their proprioceptive responses intact as they age don't have the kinds of accidents that so many older people have. You don't hear about a twenty-five-year-old falling off a curb and breaking a hip or wrist. A normal, healthy young person, even if he happens to stumble off a curb, will immediately sense that his legs are not level, and his proprioceptors will send the signals needed to let him catch his balance. Even if he should fall, warning signals from his proprioceptors will give him time to be better prepared for the fall.

If we don't use our proprioceptive ability, we lose it. A sixty- or seventy-year-old who doesn't exercise and maintain his proprioception is a candidate for falling and breaking a bone. Aerobics classes are an especially good way to tune up this ability. The great variety of movements that are a natural part of aerobics classes provide excellent training for proprioception. If you're older and are thinking, "Aerobics classes are only for younger people," think again. Proprioception is one of those things you don't know you've lost until it's too late.

Stationary Bicycle

This classic exercise device is easy for anyone to use. However, it is not weight-bearing or whole-body in nature, so fat loss is somewhat slow. On the plus side, it works well for older people, those who are pregnant or overweight or have joint problems, and beginning exercisers. It doesn't require the balance and coordination necessary for outdoor cycling, which makes it a very safe way to exercise. But, as most people who try it complain, it's boring! One way to get around that problem is to join a group class in which the instructor leads you through hills, sprints, speed paces, and flats, just as if you were in a cross-country race. For myself, I don't get bored on a stationary bicycle because it allows me to read or watch television while I exercise.

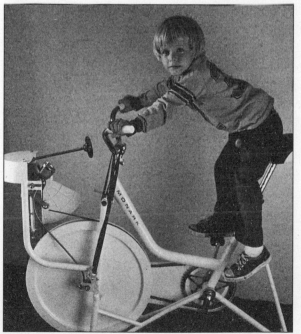

Grant Bailey, 1973

Sally Bailey

16 How Long and How Often Should I Exercise?

How long should you exercise? How should I know? I don't know how old you are, how out of shape you are, or anything else about you. For goodness sakes, get practical! Asking how long or how hard you should exercise implies that we are all the same, that one simple answer would suffice. Don't you hate it when politicians pledge to help everybody and then pass a law that fits nobody? Don't you feel bovine when you have to stand in line or, God forbid, take a number at the Department of Motor Vehicles? Nobody wants to be just a number — so don't ask for one.

When I'm interviewed for a newspaper article or a television program I'm often asked such inane questions. And I'm not the only one. The American Academy of Sports Medicine, a prestigious organization filled with highly qualified M.D.'s and Ph.D.'s, is often asked how long people should exercise. In desperation, they've come up with the suggestion that Americans should exercise three times a week for twenty minutes, as if we were all the same.

When they hear my views, most of my readers say, "At last, somebody sees me as an individual. You give me answers that let me be who I am instead of following the party line." So, rather than a rule, here's a principle:

The more muscle an exercise uses,
the less long you gotta do it!

Now you can answer "How long should I exercise?" for yourself! When you exercise, ask yourself, "How much muscle am I using?" Compare, for example, bicycling and cross-country skiing. Bicycling concentrates the effort in the thigh muscles; cross-country skiing spreads the effort through the legs, torso, and arms. What happens if you pedal hard on a bicycle? Your thighs burn. With cross-country skiing, you tend to get out of breath even before any one set of muscles starts to burn. What's the point? Bicycling uses a small number of muscles intensely, while cross-country skiing uses a large number of muscles gently.

When you feel the "burn," you are producing lactic acid, which is a sign that the muscle is burning sugar, not fat. Bicycling, which uses one set of muscles at high intensity, tends to burn less fat than cross-country skiing, which uses a lot of muscle groups at lower intensity.

The fewer muscles you use, the longer you need to exercise. If you want to shorten your exercise time, you have to find activities that incorporate lots of muscles. The more muscles you use, the greater the systemic, whole-body response and, therefore, the less long you gotta do it!

Here's another personalized principle:

If you're fit, exercise long.
If you're fat, go short but often.

In very fit people, exercising for long periods affects more than just the fat-burning enzymes. These people notice improvements in mood, sleep, and appetite control that those who exercise for only twenty or thirty minutes a day don't experience. Fat people, because their muscles tend to switch to sugar-burning more easily, don't get these improvements even if they exercise for long periods. They just get sore, cranky, and hungry. For this reason, I recommend that if

BECOME A WILD ANIMAL

A really fit person can exercise for an hour a day. When you reach the point where you can exercise for that long, you will get benefits that less fit people don't enjoy. One of them is sleep. Fit people sleep more deeply than fat people. And they go into REM — rapid eye movement or dreaming — sleep more easily. When you're really fit, you sleep like a dog. How long does it take your dog to go into REM sleep? About forty seconds, right? He comes in, makes thirty-eight turns on the rug, and flop! he's out. Pretty soon he's snoring away with his hind leg kicking. He's dreaming about the girl dog next door.

Furthermore, a dog comes out of REM sleep very quickly too. He can be sound asleep at three o'clock in the morning, but if I say, "C'mon, let's go for a run," boom! He's up and ready to go. Suppose I came into your bedroom at 3 A.M. and said, "Let's go for a run." First of all, you'd be looking for your Luger, but second, you wouldn't know where the door was! Dogs, like all very fit animals, are instantly oriented when they're awakened abruptly, an ability they need to survive in the wild. As you become more and more fit, you become more like a wild animal.

you're fat you should exercise for ten to fifteen minutes two to three times a day. As you become fitter, you should extend your exercise for longer and longer periods but also give yourself longer rests between exercise sessions.

Along the same lines, consider this:

The fatter you are the *more often* you should exercise.

I made this statement to a Boston audience: "If I were fat and needed to lose fifty pounds, I would quit my job, put my family on hold, and walk from here to Salt Lake City." That made some people mad, but most were thoughtful enough to see the point. Fat people should make exercise the most im-portant thing in their lives. They should exercise *as often as they can.* They should exercise two or three times a day, seven days a week. And their exercise should *always* be gentle enough that they never get out of breath.

Age also affects how long you should exercise:

> The older you are, the LONGER you need to exercise.
>
> BUT!
>
> You need to exercise more gently.

When your child scratches himself, how long does it take for the wound to heal? By the time you run into the house, get a Band-Aid, and run back out, the scratch is practically gone! Young people repair very quickly. We can see this clearly with a skin wound, but it's the same with all of their systems. If a child is inactive for weeks, then goes out to play for a few minutes, her muscles say, "She's exercising! Guess we'd better make some new enzymes." And they proceed to churn out hundreds of new fat-burning enzymes.

Older people, however, need to heckle their muscles into growing new fat-burning enzymes. In a twenty-year-old, ten minutes of exercise is enough to stimulate new enzyme growth, but a seventy-year-old may have to exercise upward of thirty minutes before his muscles say, "All right already! If you insist on exercising for so long I suppose I can make you a couple of extra fat-burning enzymes." But you have to be careful not to exercise too strenuously. If you exercise too hard, the muscles spend all their energy repairing damaged tissue instead of growing new tissue.

And here's another exception for older folks:

> If you're older, don't do the same exercise every day.

This ties in with what I just said about older people taking longer to repair. By varying their exercises, they can work different muscles while the previously exercised muscles are being repaired.

So! Take a number and stand in line — or think for yourself. Your body belongs to you. It's unique, it's special, and it doesn't want party-line treatment.

17 How to Get Started

First, take my two tests, the body fat test in Chapter 5 and the fitness test in Chapter 14. Coupled together, they're dynamite! There's no sense getting started if you don't know where you're going. Without a starting point, you can't measure your progress. I urge, implore, push, beg you to take my two tests.

Taking my fat test puts you light years beyond all those diet books that expect you to lose weight without having any idea whether you are losing fat or losing muscle. Don't rely on the bathroom scales to tell you that you're losing fat. To say "I used to be fat" is too vague. We need a more specific way to talk about it. If I meet you someday, I want you to be able to tell me, "I used to be thirty percent fat and now I'm down to twenty-five percent."

My fitness test will also help you keep track of your progress. Saying something like "I feel fitter now" is nice, but it's much too subjective and vague. How much fitter? How fit were you before? Using my fitness test gives you numbers so that before-and-after comparisons are real and comparisons with other people are useful. I want you to be able to tell me that you used to do a fifteen-minute mile and now you can do a twelve.

Together, the two tests put you head and shoulders above the uneducated masses who try to lose weight and get fit through trial and error and hocus-pocus.

Memorize These Rules
- Aerobic exercise requires the use of the legs and buttocks muscles to get a whole-body, systemic response.
- It has to be nonstop to be truly aerobic. You can't just walk down the street pausing to talk to everybody.
- You should not get out of breath while you do it.

If you aren't following all three of these rules, then you aren't doing aerobic exercise.

If You Can't Do It Right, Do It Often

What do I mean by this strange statement? People sometimes get too hung up on rules. They don't realize that a whole lot of "not quite aerobic" exercise can be just as good as a moderate amount of true aerobic exercise. Even though you may be breaking one of the three rules, you can still get aerobic benefit if you exercise a lot. For instance, the rule that you can't pause in the middle of your exercise would classify tennis as nonaerobic because it's a stop-and-go exercise. Nonetheless, if you play tennis for an hour or two, you can definitely increase your aerobic fitness. Your body will change just as if you had been jogging nonstop.

Remember! If you can't exercise exactly by the rules I've given you, just do a lot of it. Quantity can substitute for quality. That's why sports almost always make people fitter than strict exercise at a health club.

Don't Exercise with a Fit Friend

You can probably see the point of this one right off. If you are really fat or really out of shape, it's too hard on your body to run or bicycle at your friend's pace. Obviously, you can exercise with a fitter person if he or she doesn't try to push you or make you feel bad. I'm only telling you to be careful.

Sometimes, with the best intentions, a friend will push you too hard because the exercise is so easy for him. You end up getting injured or discouraged while your friend thinks the exercise was nothing.

Start So Slowly That People Make Fun of You

I deliberately said that in a peculiar way so you'd pay attention. There are benefits to exercising slowly. I can't emphasize this enough: *gentle exercise pays off*. If you are exercising at a slow pace, at 65 percent of your maximum heart rate, say, your body will adapt and profit from the exercise. If you're just walking, it may not seem like much to you or your friends, but at night, as you sleep, your body will say, "Boy, she doesn't exercise very hard, but she sure does a lot of it. I'd better adapt to this."

Exercise as Often as Possible

I hate cumbersome rules! Should you exercise for twenty minutes or thirty? Every day or alternate days? In the end, the rule should be to get out there and exercise as much as you possibly can. We like to see people do lots and lots of exercise.

For example, if I were fat and out of condition, I would exercise five times a day. I would find time to exercise morning, noon, and night. I might get a mini-trampoline and bounce on it in the morning when I first woke up to warm up my body. I wouldn't worry about how hard to jump, or how high, or how often. I would just bounce on the thing and have fun. Look at the three rules: a mini-trampoline uses the big muscles and doesn't get you out of breath.

I'd have a treadmill or an aerobic rider at my place of work and use it during my breaks. I'd get on it once, twice, even three times a day — again, not doing it hard, just doing it often. I'd take walks at lunch. For three months I would eat all my lunches during these walks. Some worrywart might tell you that you shouldn't eat while you exercise. Well, that's true if you're doing hard competitive exercise, but going for a brisk walk while eating a sandwich is not going to bother your stomach or your muscles. You'll probably eat more slowly, eat less, and, in the end, be better off.

In the evening I'd go for a fifteen-minute walk after dinner. All through the day I would squeeze in fifteen minutes of exercise here, ten minutes there. I wouldn't think about how many times a day I need to exercise. I would just do it whenever I could. Remember — the fatter you are, the more often you should exercise.

Don't Even Think about Distance

It doesn't matter how far you go. What matters is how many minutes a day you spend trying to change your body into a fit body. Exercise for time, not distance.

When you exercise for time only, you have two advantages. First, you don't need to find a measured course or track. All you need is a wristwatch. You can go anywhere. Second, you aren't tempted to exercise too hard because you're not trying to reach some destination. If you decide to run or cycle faster, it won't make the time go any faster. If you are shooting for a certain distance, you'll try to go faster to get it over with. But you can't hurry up time.

Somebody once remarked that we ought to match exercise minutes with the number of minutes we eat. Just think how many minutes a day you spend shoving food into your mouth! If you were to match even half of those minutes doing exercise, you would probably be fitter than a fox. Ask yourself, "Am I spending enough time each day to let my body change in a positive way?"

Cold Weather Is Not an Excuse

Why do people raise objections to exercising in the cold but leap at the chance to go skiing, snowshoeing, ice skating, ice fishing, or any one of a dozen other winter sports? As long as something is fun we don't object to the cold. We don't say, "Oh, I mustn't go skating today because the cold might be bad for me." That's a joke. Don't use cold weather as an excuse.

Rain Is Not an Excuse Either

I live in Portland, Oregon, where it rains so much that people have webs between their toes. Yet more Portlanders run than do the residents of practically any other city in the country. Running in the rain is fun! Go out, get wet, come back, and jump in the shower — it's a wonderful experience.

Some of you won't exercise in bad weather because you're afraid you'll fall on the slippery roads, or you'll catch a cold, or your hair will get ruined. Fine. Put an aerobic exercise videotape in your VCR, or get on a stationary bicycle, or go to the gym. No excuses!

Find a Sport or Make One

People who make a sport out of their exercise have a real advantage. For example, let's compare using an indoor stationary bicycle with riding a bike outdoors. In theory they should be the same. But! If you compare one hundred people who use outdoor bicycles with one hundred who use stationary bicycles, you will find that the outdoor bicyclists are much fitter, stay fitter, and usually are a lot happier.

Why is this? There are many reasons, but the most obvious is that the outdoor bicyclists put a lot more time into their exercise. If you go to the gym to use a stationary bicycle, you grit your teeth and grind out your required twenty minutes. But once you get on an outdoor bike, your inclination is to pedal much longer. You just keep going and going because it's fun. Another reason outdoor bicyclists are fitter is that they often ride with friends. They go on lots of outings just to do something with their friends. In addition, when you bicycle outdoors you need to balance the bike, negotiate turns, make sudden stops. You work your muscles more deeply and in a different way than on a stationary bicycle. Stationary bicycling concentrates most of the effort in the lower body; outdoor bicycling adds the upper-body muscles.

Try a Wind Sprint

If you're just beginning an exercise program, don't do wind sprints — or anything fast — during the first four weeks. Your exercise program should be a little bit boring at first. After a month of gentle aerobic exercise, pick one day of the week and do one or possibly two wind sprints. Wait a whole week before you do it again to make sure that you don't overdo it. (Read Chapters 20 and 21 for tips on how to get the most from wind sprints without hurting yourself.)

Forget about Calories

People ask me all the time about calories. They want to know which exercises burn the most calories. In truth, exercise doesn't burn a whole lot of calories. You'd have to run for an hour to burn off the calories in a candy bar. So stop thinking about how many calories you burn during exercise. The real reason to exercise is to change your body's chemistry, not to burn a lot of calories.

Don't Diet

Americans seem to have a mania for counting calories and going on diets. Well, take heart. I never, never want you to diet! In practice, people need to make just one dietary change: eat less fat. If you don't eat fat, you can eat a lot of food without feeling deprived. You won't feel as if you're dieting, because you aren't! Simply make the decision not to put grease on your food anymore. The simplest way to do that is to stop putting butter, margarine, mayonnaise, or any other grease on top of your food.

What a waste it is to start a good exercise program and then put a pat of oily, 100 percent vitamin-free grease on a piece of toast. There is enough fat *in* our foods without putting more fat on top of them. I've written an entire book about ways to get fat out of your diet. However, to get started, you don't need to read any more books or go to any more seminars. To start getting fit while getting rid of your body fat, do the exercises I have described and avoid fat in your diet any way you can.

Eat Often

Diets mean deprivation. I want you to do just the opposite — eat often. Fat people skip meals, fast, and try gimmicky diets, thinking that they will shed pounds. But in the end, all they do is train their bodies to exist on less and less food. If you want to train your body to be a fat-burning machine, you should eat five or six times a day, selecting foods that are low in fat and high in complex carbohydrates. Please note! I didn't say you should eat lots of food — just eat more often.

If You Have Any More Questions, Ask a Fox

That statement is a little flip. What I mean is, use common sense. If you think you are not ready to start an exercise program today because you still have too many questions, you are just kidding yourself. *Start right now.* Get out and go. Stop worrying about when to exercise, where to exercise, how long to exercise. Just do it! Would you ask a fox how long he exercises

> I don't care whether you're thirty or ninety. Get out and do some exercise, remembering that older tissues take longer to repair.

each day? Would you ask a twelve-year-old boy whether he considers it better to bike or to run? Do you tell your dog to be sure to do his aerobics at ten o'clock in the morning?

The point is, fit creatures just exercise a lot. They get out and they go. They don't worry about the time of day. If you're a morning person, exercise in the morning. If you're an evening person, exercise in the evening. You don't need someone with a Ph.D. to tell you that a certain time of day is better than any other time of day. The right time is what works for you.

Older people sometimes chide me for not addressing their special problems. I *do* address older people, and I'm addressing you now. It doesn't make any difference to me if you are thirty or ninety. Get out and do some exercise, remembering that when you are older, your tissues take longer to repair. Obey all the rules in this book, including the rule that you should go more slowly than younger people. Take it easy, stretch a little more. Just be careful. For heaven's sake, if you are seventy years old, you are supposed to be smart by now. Apply those brains to everything in this book: slow down and use your common sense!

Don't let pregnancy stop you either. After all, a pregnant fox doesn't stop exercising. Obviously, you shouldn't do exercises that bounce or jar you or put you at risk for falling. Swim, use gliding-type machines, switch from jogging to walking. Common sense tells you that this is not the time to go skiing or horseback riding.

People even worry about whether to exercise before or after a meal. Stop splitting hairs! If you're one of those people who throws up if you exercise right after eating, then don't do it. Stop asking nitpicking questions. Just get out and exercise.

Repeat to Yourself While Exercising

"I'm not burning a lot of calories while I'm exercising, but my body is changing into a better butter-burning machine. The purpose of my exercise is to change my chemistry."

If you keep repeating that to yourself, you won't fall into the trap of wondering what to eat, how many calories you are burning during the exercise, or whether you are doing it exactly right. It doesn't matter. Say to yourself, "I need a tune-up, and that's why I'm exercising." How your body repairs, changes, and improves *after* exercise is what matters.

Give Yourself a Break

Exercise is useless if you don't take time to recover from it. If you wake up in the morning tired instead of energetic, you need a break. If you're grumpy instead of cheerful, take some time off! When exercise becomes a chore instead of an anticipated playtime, you need to rest. Take a day or two off. Take a week. It doesn't mean you're lazy. Top-notch athletes are as serious about their rest and recovery as they are about their exercise. They know they will actually perform better after a couple of days of rest.

18 The *Fastest* Way to Improve Fitness

The fastest way to improve fitness is to do hard, intense exercise. Whoa! I've just spent all this time giving you the reasons why you should do gentle, low-key aerobic exercise, and now I tell you that intense exercise raises fitness. What's going on?

There are three ways to get fitter: you can exercise longer; you can exercise more often; or you can exercise harder. Unquestionably, no argument, exercising harder gives the fastest results. But I'll bet you've never heard that before. Your aerobics teacher has certainly never said that. I never said it in my earlier books. Why not? The reason is obvious. You can get hurt if you exercise hard. Better to teach people to exercise gently and get fit slowly.

So what should you do? Exercise gently all the time and take forever to get fitter? Or exercise intensely but chance getting injured? There is a solution. There are ways to add intensity to your exercise program WITHOUT getting hurt. It is possible to "trick" your muscles into thinking they are doing intense work without really overworking them. Let me show you how.

$\Rightarrow$

Covert Bailey's Four Food Groups of Good Exercise

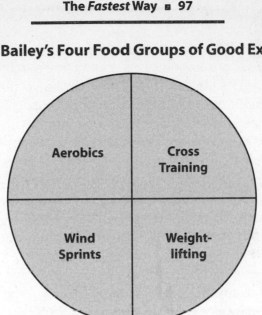

Get a balanced diet of good exercise.

The "Four Food Groups" of Exercise

Everyone has heard of the four food groups. The premise of the system is simple — you should eat a balanced diet. Eating only one kind of food all the time is not smart; you won't get all the essential vitamins, minerals, and other nutrients.

Doing the same exercise over and over isn't smart either. It's better to balance your exercises, just as you balance your diet. At the end of every week you should be able to look back and say, "I did an exercise from each of Covert's four exercise groups."

The four essential weekly exercise activities are:

- Aerobic exercise
- Cross training
- Wind sprints
- Weightlifting

What is cross training? Simply put, it means alternating between two (or sometimes three) different aerobic exercises rather than sticking to one. You may argue that the first group, aerobic exercise, and the second group, cross training, are both aerobic, so why make it sound like a whole new thing? I want to be sure that people visualize the second group as essential for smart exercising, for there is a lot more to cross training than first appears (see Chapter 19).

The third "food group" of exercise is wind sprints. Many people think you do sprints simply by going fast, then slow, then fast, then slow. They don't understand the subtleties involved. For example, how fast should you go, and how slow? How long should the fast part be? Let's say you want to add wind sprints to your daily jog. Should you run as fast as you can, going at your absolute maximum? Should you sprint for a few seconds or for several minutes?

Here's another thing to think about. Not only can you vary the sprint part, but you can vary the recovery part afterward. After you go back to the exercise you were doing before the sprint, how long should you exercise before you do another sprint? You can see that wind sprints are more than just fast, slow, fast, slow. You can manipulate a number of variables, depending on your goals and the kind of athletics you're interested in. The right combination can make you a faster sprinter or a better basketball player or, if your main goal is to lose fat, a better butter-burner. In Chapter 20 I'll describe how to do wind sprints in a way that adds intensity to your exercise program but doesn't wear you out.

The fourth group of exercise is weightlifting. If you have never lifted weights, please don't tune me out. I can show you how to make it fun and comfortable. My reason for making it one of the four essential exercises has little to do with making your muscles larger or getting stronger. Instead, I focus on the physiological effects that occur AFTER weightlifting. Wonderful changes in metabolism take place during the forty-eight-hour recovery period (see Chapter 22).

If you want to get the most out of your exercise time — if you want to get fit fast and want your body to learn how to burn fat — then exercise from each of the four food groups every week.

19 Cross Training

You can raise your fitness more quickly by doing two different exercises rather than sticking to one. If you're an everyday jogger, you'll be better off jogging only four days a week and bicycling on the other one or two days. If you are an everyday swimmer, you'll be better off doing an exercise on land one or two days a week. In other words, do two different aerobic exercises for maximum aerobic benefit. Now let me tell you why and how to do it.

Doing one aerobic exercise will make you fit, BUT! alternating between two exercises will make you fit *faster* — and with less chance of injury. Remember, *intensity* increases fitness fastest. If you do just one exercise, you have to do it more and more intensely to get improvements. But if you switch to another exercise without increasing your intensity, your muscles will react as if you *were* working harder. Alternating between two exercises at lower intensity tricks the muscles into making fitness adaptations as if you were doing one exercise at ever-increasing intensity.

Suppose, for example, that you've been jogging for several weeks. The fat-burning enzymes inside your muscles have grown to a certain size and number to handle the exercise, but now they've stopped growing because they've reached a level that competently handles the amount of exercise you're doing. When this happens, you've hit a "plateau." Your fat loss seems to slow down. You're sort of in a rut. So what do you do? Jog faster, right? This wakes up the fat-burning enzymes: "Hey! She's running faster! We need to hire on more workers!" Pretty soon, your fat loss picks up again and everything is fine *until* . . . you reach the next plateau. So once again you pick up your speed. And again you get results, but at some point you're not going to want to — or be able to — run faster. At that point, many people say the heck with this!

In an earlier chapter I described the fat-burning enzymes as lazy. They really don't want to work very hard. They won't burn fat unless you're exercising gently. If you start exercising so hard that you get out of breath, the fat-burning enzymes will cop out and turn the energy-providing job over to the sugar-burning enzymes. However, as long as the exercise is aerobic, the fat-burning enzymes will work. If the work gets harder but is still aerobic, they hire on new workers. If you switch to a different exercise but do it at a gentle aerobic intensity, your muscles THINK they're working harder, so they grow more fat-burning enzymes.

You can see now why I started you out right away with two different exercises in my basic fitness program (described at the end of Chapter 14). I could have told you to do just one exercise, but by doing two, you'll build fat-burning enzymes more quickly. After about six months you may reach a plateau with these exercises. Instead of exhausting yourself by doing them faster and harder, simply select two new exercises and continue to exercise at an easy, moderate level. You've added intensity without getting hurt.

The beauty of cross training is that you can add intensity to your exercise program *without* exercising harder, *without* exercising longer, and *without* exercising more often.

Think about this. If you do just one exercise day after day, one set of muscles gets very, very efficient at burning fat. But

---

HOW DOES CROSS TRAINING INCREASE INTENSITY?

In cross training, we make muscles move in ways they aren't used to. Since these muscles are not accustomed to the new exercise, the work required is more intense for them. By switching from one moderate activity to another moderate activity, you can fool muscles into thinking they're exercising more intensely.

---

other muscles right next to them may not be burning fat as well. By doing a different exercise, you train more and more muscles to become better fat-burners. Both the fat person and the fit person can profit from this. The fat person acquires more fat-burning enzymes; the fit person can exercise longer and harder during sports. Think of the fun athletes have when they are able to play and run for hours without getting out of breath!

Cross training also gives you greater coordination and balance by training more sets of nerves. There are long-distance runners who look like gazelles on the racetrack yet are awkward at other sports. Die-hard runners would do themselves a favor if they added a second, different exercise to their repertoire.

Well, then, you ask, would it be better to do four or five different exercises instead of two? No, that doesn't seem to work as well. You need to do an exercise at least twice a week for your body to recognize it as an activity you do all the time and make the necessary systemic and neurological adjustments to adapt to it. There's nothing wrong with doing a variety of exercises, but the greatest fitness adaptations seem to occur with two or, at the most, three different aerobic exercises.

It's a shame that older people don't make better use of cross training. As you get into your sixties and beyond, it's harder to retain muscle mass. Older people lose muscle more easily because they can't exercise as vigorously as younger people and because it takes longer to build and repair muscle. Cross training offers older folks a way to maintain muscle mass and strength without getting exhausted.

Choosing Your Cross-Training Exercises

Combine an outdoor exercise with an indoor exercise so that you have no excuse to avoid exercise on bad-weather days. The indoor exercise could be aerobics classes, an exercise videotape, or an exercise machine.

Choose exercises that use a variety of muscles; that way, lots of muscles learn to work aerobically instead of just a few. For example, swimming combined with walking uses practically every muscle in the body. Elite athletes who train for specific

---

WHAT DO I MEAN BY INTENSITY?

I worry that people may quote me out of context — "Covert Bailey says you have to do intense exercise if you want to get fit." If that is all they say, their friends will think that intensity means going as fast as they possibly can. Not true! I've just showed you how to add intensity without exercising harder simply by switching exercises. To your muscles, this change seems like added intensity. In the next chapter, I will describe another way to add intensity by going just a little faster for just a short time.

Intensity is a relative term — it means pushing yourself beyond what's comfortable. I am trying to show you how to add little bits of intensity WITHOUT getting hurt. If you tell a friend, "Covert Bailey says you've got to exercise intensely," be sure to explain the rest, or you're not helping your friend.

competitive sports, however, should select a cross-training exercise that is similar to their main exercise; they need to train specific muscles to work aerobically at very high, very intense levels of effort.

If you need to lose fat, choose a "let's get moving" activity, such as walking, jogging, or skiing (outdoor or machine) and combine it with a whole-body activity such as using an aerobic rider or stair climber or rowing (outdoors or with a machine). Moving your weight around from one spot to another burns fat more quickly than staying in one place jumping rope or bouncing on a trampoline or sitting on a bicycle.

If you are pregnant, combine swimming (or water aerobics) with stationary bicycling, machine rowing, an aerobic rider, or some other whole-body exercise machine. Avoid bouncing or jarring exercises.

If you're older, pick exercises that use different sets of muscles, so that one set can repair while you exercise the other. Swimming, which uses the upper-body muscles more than any other aerobic exercise, is an excellent cross-training choice. It's not the fastest way to burn fat, so couple it with a land exercise.

As you age, your muscles are more likely to stiffen up after exercise, which increases your chance of injury. Here again, swimming (or an aerobic water activity) is the answer. Nobody ever says, "Boy, I sprained my ankle swimming!" Exercise in the water can be very intense, but it doesn't have the pounding and jarring associated with other forms of hard exercise. If you don't have access to a swimming pool you could try one of the machines I call "dry-land swimming machines" because you can't get hurt on them. For example, the HealthRider (and other aerobic riders) uses all the muscles in the body yet puts stress on none of them, just as if you were swimming.

If you're a die-hard runner unable to stand the thought of missing a single day of running, add a sport similar to running, such as cross-country skiing or in-line skating.

If you're a tennis lover (or enjoy some other nonaerobic sport), make that sport your main activity, but add twenty minutes of jogging or cycling on alternate days. As I said earlier, you can get fit doing nonaerobic sports. On a per-minute basis they're not as effective in raising fitness as aerobic exercise, but what the heck? If you love the sport, you'll do a lot of it, right? And a lot of something you love works much better than twenty minutes of something you hate.

20 Wind Sprints

To an athlete, "wind sprint" is a familiar term, one that means going very fast. But it's the first word — WIND — that should be emphasized, because it's "getting winded" that makes wind sprints work. It might have been easier to explain this technique if I had made up a new name for it, such as "the Get Winded Exercise." Athletes have to go very fast to get winded. Out-of-shape people can get winded just from walking.

Right away you should see that getting winded is a glaring contradiction to everything I've written up to this point. I've told you over and over to exercise slowly and gently so that your muscles burn fat instead of sugar. I've told you not to get out of breath when you exercise. Now I'm going to recommend it.

It is true that aerobic exercise burns fat, but if you're out of shape your current level of exercise is not strenuous enough to burn great quantities of fat. It would be great if you could run and play the way young kids do, burning fat the way they do, but you can't do that anymore.

Compare a very fit athlete with someone who hasn't exercised in years. The athlete can run a mile in five minutes — *without getting out of breath.* He is aerobic, burning fat the whole time. The out-of-shape person might cover only one-quarter of a mile in five minutes. The athlete would burn forty fat calories in his five minutes, while the out-of-shape person would burn only about fifteen. So the out-of-shape guy would have to jog for twelve minutes to burn the amount of fat the athlete burns in five. The out-of-shape guy just doesn't have the quality or quantity of fat-burning enzymes in his muscles. This notion may sound silly, but if you are planning to gain ten pounds over the Christmas holidays, you should build lots of fat-burning enzymes in your muscles beforehand so you can burn off the fat quickly when the festivities are over!

If you want to become a person who burns LOTS of fat during aerobic exercise, then you have to raise the level at which you exercise. Doing little bursts of "get winded" exercise in the middle of your regular aerobic exercise session is what raises that level.

A wind sprint is a short burst of higher-intensity exercise in the middle of low-intensity exercise. I like to use jogging as my example, but you can apply the technique to any aerobic exercise. Jog at your regular aerobic pace for approximately ten minutes until you are breathing deeply but comfortably. Now break into a faster jog for twenty to forty seconds. After that time, don't stop, just go back to your regular aerobic pace. You'll be out of breath and want to stop, but make yourself keep jogging. For a minute or so your breathing will be hard, but then it will return to its regular deep, comfortable, aerobic level. In essence, you're forcing your body to recover under stress; that is, it must recover while you continue to exercise.

If you read the last paragraph carefully, you'll notice that I didn't tell you to do a breakneck run. I just want you to jog a little faster than usual. If you are bicycling, you should pedal a little harder but not as hard as possible. The same rule applies to any aerobic exercise you do. When you "sprint" during the exercise, do it slightly harder rather than going all out.

That little sprint in the middle of your exercise allows you to add intensity without injuring yourself. You don't have to go superfast. You don't have to do it superlong. Just do a little sprint, something that makes you breathe harder, so that when you go back to the pace you were at before, whatever that comfortable pace was, it's not as comfortable as it was. That's the key to wind sprints. It's not how hard or fast you do them, it's the *recovery after the sprint* that makes you get fit fast. The fat-burning enzymes say, "It's bad enough that we have to grow when she does aerobic exercise — now she does these little sprints; we're going to have to grow even faster."

When I was young I thought I had to do a sprint as hard and as fast as possible, that there was something magical about pushing myself to the wall. I now know that the magical part of the wind sprint is the recovery from it. I urge you, don't run extremely hard, don't run at full speed. Just increase your

---

WHAT DO I MEAN BY INTENSITY?

(Yes, I'm Repeating Myself)

I'm still worried that people will interpret intensity to mean hard, exhausting exercise. Using wind sprints to add intensity means exercising just a little bit harder than usual for just a few moments. Let's say you are terribly out of shape and fifty pounds overfat. Slow walking is your fastest comfortable exercise. In the middle of your walk you go up a short hill, which makes you puff a little. The uphill stretch is not hard enough or long enough to exhaust you or make you gasp, but it's enough extra effort to make you glad to reach the top. That little hill represents the level of intensity I'm talking about. Sprinting madly up the hill as if it were an emergency would be too intense, too exhausting for you. An Olympic athlete, however, would have to race up a much steeper hill to add intensity to her comfortable run.

effort enough so that you get a little winded. After the sprint I want you to jog *at the same pace* as before the sprint, only now that pace won't be as comfortable. You've actually added intensity in two ways, haven't you? The sprint itself adds intensity, and the pace that was comfortable *before* the sprint is intense to your muscles *afterward*. To raise fitness and thus burn more fat, you must force your body to recover under stress. If you do wind sprints the way I've described, you can raise your fitness level very fast WITHOUT getting hurt.

If you're fat, you may be thinking, "That wind-sprint stuff is for fit people." Not so! You can benefit from wind sprints just as much as the athletes do. The only difference is the intensity of your sprint. Let's say a slow walk is all you can do without getting out of breath. It takes you twenty minutes to walk a mile aerobically. People watching you from a distance would think you're just out for a casual stroll. If you broke into a run, you'd probably feel embarrassed. But if you do wind sprints the way I've described, no one will think you look silly, because all you'll be doing is walking fast for twenty to forty seconds. Just walk along at your comfortable aerobic pace and then walk fast for the distance between two telephone poles or the length of two houses. Get moving fast enough that you're out of breath for twenty to forty seconds, then drop back to your original pace. Sure, it may not look like you're doing much, but your body will respond to the stress just as an athlete's body would respond. I've said it three times — you don't have to sprint superhard or superlong for it to be effective. It's not the intensity of the sprint that changes your body. It's the intensity of the recovery. You must force your body to recuperate while it is under stress.

Athletes do wind sprints without thinking about it. Young kids do wind sprints all the time. Watch four or five kids playing Frisbee. They sort of hop around, jogging easily as they toss the Frisbee back and forth. But once in a while the Frisbee sails over someone's head so that he has to run to catch it. The kids unconsciously add intensity in the middle of what looks like gentle play. By mixing low-level exercise with high-level, sprintlike activity, they get very fit. Their low-level exercise burns lots of fat. Their high-level activity raises their fitness.

When your level of fitness is raised, fat-burning increases in two ways. First, a fit person who can exercise at high intensity *without getting out of breath* burns more fat than someone who does the same exercise at lower intensity. Second, as you become fitter, you can do more activities without getting out of breath. In effect, becoming fit means becoming like a kid again. You do lots of exercise without realizing you're even exercising. And all these "unconscious" bouts of more intense activity are great for burning fat. Wind sprints raise your level of fitness so that you can exercise more strenuously and burn ever-increasing amounts of fat, yet your body doesn't perceive the higher level of exercise as more intense, so you don't get hurt.

Covert's Rules for Wind Sprints

- Sprint easy, recover hard.
- You don't have to sprint to do wind sprints — you just have to get winded.
- It's not the intensity of the sprint that matters — it's the intensity of the recovery.

21 How Fast Should You Do Wind Sprints?

People have trouble figuring out how fast or hard to do wind sprints. I've said that they shouldn't be done very fast or hard, but what exactly does that mean?

You can do wind sprints during any exercise — bicycling, rowing, swimming, whatever — but the easiest way for me to teach you the correct intensity is to have you do them while walking or jogging (or running, if you're really fit).

The intensity of your wind sprint is determined by your aerobic pace. (If you don't know your aerobic pace, refer back to Chapter 14.) The table below tells you how fast your sprint should be based on your aerobic pace. I've also included miles-per-hour speeds for those who have access to a treadmill. I've found that a treadmill is an excellent way to get used to doing wind sprints without overdoing them.

Once you get used to the intensity needed to sprint when you walk or jog, you can then apply that same intensity of breathing and effort to any other aerobic exercise.

Wind-Sprint Training

If you do wind sprints the way I've described, you will raise your fitness level and increase fat-burning. Wind sprints work for anyone, regardless of their fitness level. For those of you who are into competitive sports, there are ways to further

How Fast Should You Do Wind Sprints?

If your aerobic pace* is (min./mile)	Then your aerobic exercise is	And your wind-sprint speed should be	Your treadmill pace is (mph)	And your treadmill sprint should be (mph)
5–6	Fast run	Sprint	10	12–15
7–8	Moderate run	Fast run	7.5	9.0
9–10	Fast jog	Slow run	6.0	7.0
11–12	Moderate jog	Fast jog	5.0	6.0
13–15	Fast walk	Moderate jog	4.0	5.0
16–18	Moderate walk	Slow jog	3.5	4.5
19–20	Slow walk	Fast walk	3.0	4.0
More than 20	Do not add wind sprints to your program until you can walk a mile in 20 minutes without getting out of breath.			

*Aerobic pace means the speed at which you can run consecutive, nonstop miles without getting out of breath.

tweak your wind-sprint training. The first box on page 113 is for the 98 percent of us who just want to be lean and fit; the second is for the 2 percent who want to have an edge over their rivals.

Wind-Sprint Training for Regular People

Intensity of sprint: Moderately hard; faster than your normal pace but NOT all out. (If you're walking, then your sprint is a jog. If you're jogging, then your sprint is a run. And if you're running, then your sprint is really a sprint.)

Duration of sprint: 20–40 seconds

Duration of recovery: If you do more than one sprint, do not start the next one until you are back to pre-sprint breathing level.

How often? Once a week during one of your regular aerobic workouts. (You may reduce your total exercise time that day by 5–10 minutes.)

How many during 20-minute workout? 1–5. For the first two weeks, do just one sprint during your exercise. After that, add one sprint each week until you can do 2–5 sprints during a 20-minute workout.

Wind-Sprint Training for Athletes

Type of athlete	Intensity of sprint	Duration of sprint	Duration of recovery	How often?	How many during a 30-min. workout?
Short-distance (sprinting, weightlifting)	High (95–100% of mhr*)	10–20 sec.	Three times as long as sprint	2–3 times per week	20–40
Middle-distance; stop-and-go (basketball, racquetball, soccer)	Moderately high (85–90% of mhr*)	1–2 min.	Twice as long as sprint	1–2 times per week	5–10
Long-distance (marathon runner)	Moderate (80–85% of mhr*)	3–5 min.	Half as long as sprint	Once a week	4–6

*Maximum heart rate

Here's What I Want You to Add to Your Program

Continue doing four twenty-minute aerobic and cross-training sessions a week, but!

Add wind sprints* to one of your sessions, as follows:

- Warm up at a speed slower than your usual aerobic pace for at least five minutes.
- Exercise at your aerobic pace for five to ten minutes.
- Speed up to a moderately hard pace for twenty to forty seconds, but don't go all out. If you're walking, your sprint is a jog. If you're jogging, your sprint is a run. And if you're running, your sprint is really a sprint.
- Return to your pre-sprint pace (you will now be breathing hard as you recover from the sprint).
- When you are once again breathing deeply but comfortably, do another sprint.
- In the beginning add only one or two sprints; as you get fitter add up to five sprints.
- After your last sprint, continue exercising at your aerobic pace for at least five minutes, then cool down for at least another five minutes at a speed slower than your aerobic pace.

*Do not add wind sprints to your program until you can walk a mile in 20 minutes without getting out of breath. Do not add wind sprints to your program until you have been on an aerobic exercise program for at least four weeks.

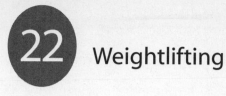

22 Weightlifting

Weightlifting is not aerobic — ever! You may think you're breathing aerobically when you lift weights, but believe me, no matter how deeply you breathe, you can't supply enough oxygen to the muscle to make it aerobic: the demand is simply too intense. To your muscles, weightlifting is not gentle exercise and is thus totally anaerobic, so fat-burning shuts down. Muscles burn only sugar during weightlifting, so they produce lactic acid, which causes that sensation called the "burn."

In spite of this fact, plenty of people have lost body fat by weightlifting. How come? And why do I recommend it for weight loss? I have two reasons. First, weightlifting strengthens your muscles, so you can perform your aerobic exercise more intensely without becoming anaerobic. Think about what that means. Stronger muscles derived through anaerobic weightlifting let you burn more fat during your aerobic exercise because you don't get out of breath so quickly.

Second, and more important, the recovery phase of weightlifting has a profound impact on the fat-burning enzymes. You may feel calm and relaxed after lifting weights, but your fat-burning enzymes are working like crazy to repair the damage. One of their biggest

> If you feel the burn, then your muscles are using sugar for fuel, not fat.

jobs is to replace the sugar that was used by the sugar-burning enzymes.

Our muscles have a very strong physiological drive to replace muscle sugar (glycogen) in order to be prepared for emergencies. They say, "We need to restock our sugar supplies — and we need it *now!*" Where is the sugar going to come from? You can't just dump sugar into your body and expect to store it in your muscles. The muscles have to change the sugar into a special form called glycogen, which is easy to store. And to do that, the muscles need energy. After exercise, the fat-burning enzymes burn fat to produce energy, which is then used by the muscles to store sugar. Our bodies break down fat supplies to build up the sugar supplies.

Restoring sugar requires a lot of energy, which means that lots of calories are burned. And *all* of this energy must be supplied by the fat-burning enzymes. Now you can see why I want you to lift weights. When sugar is drained from a muscle (and the intensity of weightlifting quickly drains it), it's up to the fat-burning enzymes to see that the sugar is replenished. Fat isn't burned *during* weightlifting, but a *lot* of fat is burned afterward.

Replacing sugar isn't the only job that has to be done after weightlifting. Damaged fibers in the muscles have to be repaired, and that takes energy, which is produced by the fat-burning enzymes. Weightlifting also stimulates the muscles to get bigger, and muscle growth demands even more energy.

What I'm saying in about ten different ways is that weightlifting stimulates metabolism and fat-burning. The heat that emanates from your muscles after you lift weights is not residual heat from the work you've just done. That heat is lost in seconds. Instead, what you're feeling is the heat of metabolism during the recovery *after* weightlifting. Weightlifters sometimes get mad when I say that weightlifting doesn't burn off fat. But you can see now that weightlifting burns lots of fat for metabolism during the hours, or even days, of recovery.

> Fat is not burned *during* weightlifting.
> BUT!
> Lots of fat is burned during the *recovery* from weightlifting.

If you recall, the key to wind sprints was not the sprints themselves but the recovery afterward. The same is true for weightlifting. Your main focus should be on the benefits inherent in the recovery instead of the actual lifting of weights. Many people lift weights to get bigger muscles, but that's not my concern here. The reason I include weightlifting in my "four food groups" of exercise is that it puts a tremendous demand on the fat burning enzymes during recovery, and that has a tremendous effect on fat loss.

Now, with metabolism in mind rather than body building, we can approach the exercise in a very different way from a typical weightlifting program. With my program you don't have to lift heavy weights. You don't have to "max out." You don't have to work each and every muscle. In fact, you don't even have to use weights! Let's go to the next chapter to learn how to do it.

23 Covert's Home Weightlifting Program

Everyone knows what a push-up is. But what are you pushing when you do one? You're pushing your own weight, aren't you? If you're a 150-pound guy, then you're pushing part of that 150 pounds. In gyms, people do push-ups upside down; that is, they lie on their backs and push up a barbell. The exercise is called a bench press instead of a push-up. You can either lie on your back and push a barbell up or turn over and push your weight up. The two exercises are not exactly the same, but the point is that push-ups are a form of weightlifting.

Sit-ups are another way to lift weight using your body as the weight. Doing sit-ups, or crunches, while lying on your back uses muscles in the abdomen to lift the shoulders, upper trunk, and head. You're lifting a very heavy weight with a relatively small set of muscles. Any time you lift a big weight with a small muscle, you are weightlifting.

I've designed a weightlifting program you can do at home using your own body so that you don't have to buy weights or join a gym. It's not intended for experienced weightlifters — it's a starter program.

Covert's Home Weightlifting Program (No Barbells Required)

Push-Ups

The push-up is a good exercise to start with because it's easy to adapt to your own strength. If you are really heavy and out of shape, do a wall push-up: stand about two feet away from a wall with your feet apart and hands flat on the wall. Bend your elbows so your body falls toward the wall. Then slowly straighten your arms, pushing your body away from the wall while keeping the effort in your chest and shoulders. The weaker you are, the closer to the wall you should stand.

When you get strong enough, you can progress to push-ups on the floor on your hands and knees. If you are fairly athletic, you should bypass this position and do the classic

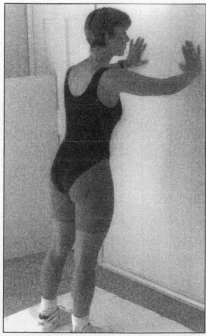

push-ups from your toes, as shown in all those army training movies. Some people are so strong that even that position is not challenging enough, so they put their feet up on a chair. The higher you put your feet, the more of your body you're lifting with your arms and the more the push-up resembles a bench press with a barbell.

Chest: Push-Ups
Level 1: Wall push-off. Start with feet about 24 inches from wall. To increase difficulty, move farther away.

Sally Bailey

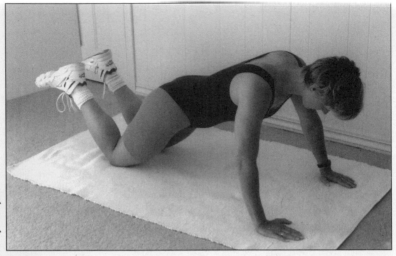

Sally Bailey

Level 2: Bent-knee push-up. Moving hands closer together or farther apart works different muscles.

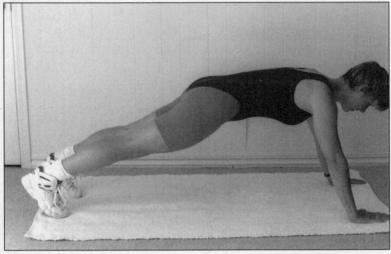

Sally Bailey

Level 3: Straight-leg push-up. Keep feet 10–15 inches apart. To increase difficulty, elevate feet on stool.

Tips: Keep back flat, not arched; keep arms bent, never locked straight; place hands slightly farther apart than shoulder width.

Squats

For your lower body — thighs, buttocks, calves — do squats. If you do them with no weights, it won't seem like much exercise until you learn to do them right. Stand about a foot in front of a chair and squat in such a way that your rear end sticks out and you almost tip over backward. Lower yourself until your buttocks touch the chair, then stand up again. Keep the lower part of your legs, from knees to feet, absolutely straight up and down. Most people doing squats allow their lower legs to lean forward so their knees project over their toes. Your knees should be in line with your toes, keeping the lower legs vertical. In order to do that you really have to stick your fanny out. It's a funny-looking exercise, but it's one of

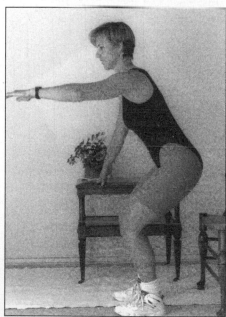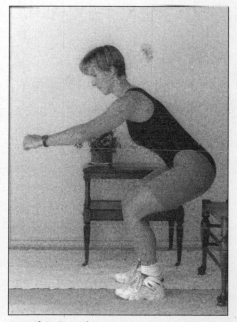

Buttocks/Legs: Squats
Level 1: Squat using table assist.

Level 2: Regular squat.

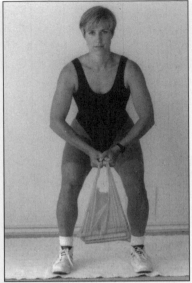

Sally Bailey

the best for strengthening your lower body. If you do squats slowly, they are a pretty intense exercise even without weights and even for people who are used to gyms and heavy barbells. Squats work the thighs and buttocks — the biggest muscles you've got. Now you're really going to get the metabolic after-effects of weightlifting.

Level 3: Squat with added weight.

Tips: Place feet shoulder-width apart. Squat as if you were going to sit down in a chair. Just when you reach the edge, stand back up. Reach hands out in front for balance. Caution! Don't let your knees extend in front of your feet.

Sit-Ups

For your midsection, do crunch-type sit-ups. Lie on your back with your knees bent, feet flat on the floor. Keeping your back flat, raise your upper body just four or five inches. This is a very subtle movement that concentrates all your effort in the abdominal muscles. If you try to raise your body too high, you're using your hips more than your abdominal muscles. If you're a beginner, you should reach your arms between your legs or clasp them across your chest. If you're moderately fit, you can clasp your hands behind your neck. And if you're very fit, you may want to hold a weight on your chest or do sit-ups from an inclined position, with your feet elevated above your head.

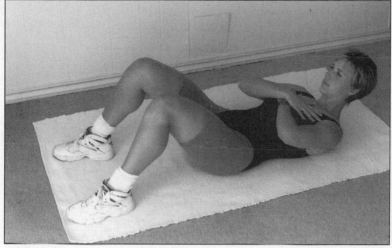

Sally Bailey

Midsection: Crunch Sit-Ups
Level 1: Crunch with arms across chest. Keep neck relaxed.

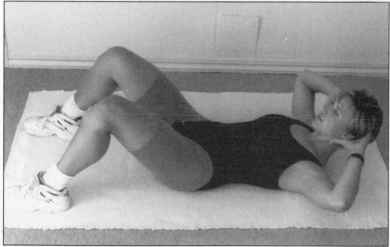

Sally Bailey

Level 2: Regular crunch sit-up. Rest head lightly in hands. Don't pull on neck or head. Keep elbows out to sides.

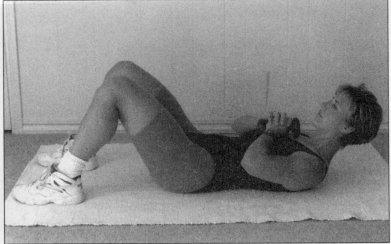

Sally Bailey

Level 3: Crunch with added weight. Keep weight high on chest. Tips: This is a very small movement — you aren't trying to touch your knees. Look up toward the ceiling.

Dips

I include dips in my home program even though they don't work a major muscle, only the small triceps on the back of the arm. But that's an area that gets flabby very easily as we get older, especially in women. To do them, sit on a chair with your feet flat on the floor. Scoot forward on the chair, moving your feet forward as you do so, and put the heels of your hands on the edge of the chair beside your buttocks. Take your weight onto your hands and arms by lifting your buttocks off the chair. Keeping your knees bent, slowly lower your body in front of the chair by bending your elbows. Then raise your body back up again. You may have to have someone hold the chair so it doesn't tip or topple over.

Beginners may be able to lift themselves up and down only three or four inches and may cheat a little by using their leg muscles. As you get stronger you can stretch your feet out more and also let yourself down farther so that the muscles on the backs of your arms get more of a workout. If you're very strong, you can stretch your legs straight out in front or put them on a stool so that even more weight is supported by the backs of your arms.

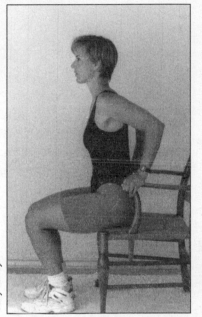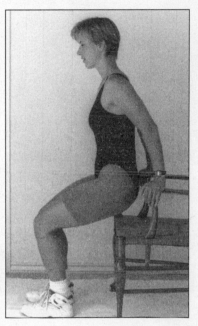

Sally Bailey

Back of Arms: Dips
Level 1: Sit-to-stand dip. Use chair arms to push yourself up and out of chair.

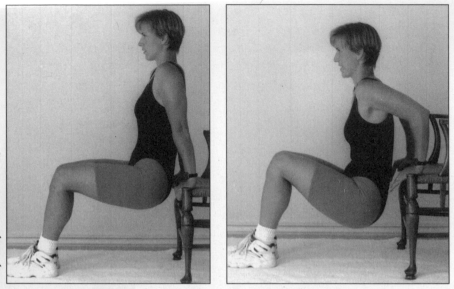

Sally Bailey

Level 2: Bent-knee dip. Finger tips face forward. Place feet a minimum of 24 inches away from chair. Keep rear end close to chair.

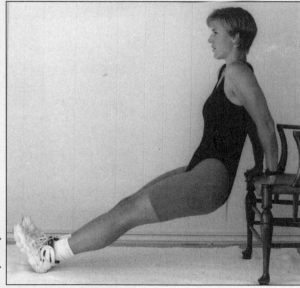

Sally Bailey

Level 3: Straight-leg dip. Fingers forward and legs straight, with slight bend in knees.

Tips: Keep the focus on your arms. It's easy to cheat and let your legs do the work. The farther your feet are from the chair, the harder the exercise.

My home weightlifting program is designed to:

• Safely add intensity to your exercise regimen.
• Slow down or prevent loss of muscle due to normal aging.
• Increase body awareness and "muscle sense."
• Speed up metabolism through repair and recuperation.

Keep in mind that this is not a muscle-building program but rather a muscle *maintenance* program. Those who want bigger muscles should use machines or free weights. My program has no "advanced" level, for that would require lifting more weight than your body alone.

People who know a lot about weightlifting may point out that these exercises don't work all the muscles of the body, but I've selected them for specific reasons. I've combined large and small muscle groups because I want you to get a twofold response. First, the squats and push-ups use major muscles and therefore stimulate those physiological after-effects I discussed in the last chapter. And second, I want you to develop muscle awareness. The sit-ups and dips use smaller muscles, which fatigue easily, so you learn very

Covert's Home Weightlifting Program

Category	What to do	How many? beginner/intermediate	Major muscles/ auxiliary muscles used
Chest	Push-ups	1 set /2–3 sets (8 –12 reps per set)	**Chest, back**/arms, abdominal muscles, shoulders
Buttocks/legs	Squats	1 set /2–3 sets (15 reps per set)	**Buttocks, hamstrings, thighs**/calves
Midsection	Crunches	10–15 /20 –30	**Abdominal muscles**
Backs of arms	Dips	1 set /2 –3 sets (8 –12 reps per set)	**Triceps**/back, shoulders, abdominal muscles

quickly what a sore muscle feels like. A key ingredient in muscle awareness is having a sense of where the muscle is. When a muscle is sore, you know EXACTLY where it is!

You've Never Weightlifted? Here Are Some Tips!

- *The magic numbers are 8 through 12.* Find a weight (or a position, if you are using your body as the weight) that you can lift 8–12 times before you get tired or feel the burn. If you can lift more than 12 times, you need a heavier weight. If you can't lift at least 8 times, you need a lighter weight.

- *Doing 8–12 repetitions is called a set.* I recommend that beginners do one or two sets, gradually increasing to three or four.

- *Work the large muscles first.* Small muscles fatigue quickly. When they get exhausted they can't assist the large muscles. So! work the large muscles first (chest, back, shoulders, thighs) and the smaller muscles last (arms, calves, abdominal muscles).

- *Focus on the muscle being worked.* Beginners often throw their entire body into a movement instead of concentrating on specific muscles. For example, if you're doing curls to work the biceps, don't thrust your torso into the lift. Keep the upper body still and concentrate all the work in the muscles of the upper arm. If you find you have to thrust your torso to complete a lift, then the weight you are using is too heavy.

- *Remember to breathe!* This sounds silly, but beginners often hold their breath during lifting, which can cause a sharp rise in blood pressure. It doesn't matter whether you inhale or exhale during the lift; you decide which feels more comfortable. Just remember to do it!

- *Wait 48 hours between sessions.* Your muscles need about 48 hours to repair after weightlifting. If you don't give your muscles time to recover, you won't get the beneficial metabolic effects.

Muscle Awareness

People who don't exercise, especially if they're also overweight, tend to trip and fall more often than fit people, who are able to catch themselves even if they do trip. Overweight people think that they fall just because they're overweight, when in fact, they do so because they don't have muscle awareness.

One of the reasons I include weightlifting in my "four food groups" of exercise is that I want you to develop muscle sense. For example, the simple dips I recommend in my home program are almost totally dependent on the muscles in the back of the arm. It's easy to build lactic acid in them and experience next-day soreness. You learn very quickly where those muscles are.

I believe that if older folks took fifteen minutes of their day to do my weightlifting program, their gain in muscle

Covert Bailey's Four Food Groups of Exercise
Recommended Weekly Allowances

Category	What to do	How long?	How often?
Aerobic exercise	Aerobic exercise #1	20–30 min.	2 times per week
Cross training	Aerobic exercise #2	20–30 min.	1 time per week
Wind sprints	Increase speed or intensity during aerobic exercise #1 or #2	1–5 sprints (20–40 sec. each)	1 time per week during aerobic exercise #1 or #2 (shorten this session to 15–20 minutes)
Weightlifting	Covert's Home Weightlifting Program	15–25 min.	2 times per week

awareness would cause a significant drop in those classic accidents of old age such as broken hips and fractured wrists. In following my home weightlifting program, remember to:
- Make movements slow and strong.
- Breathe!
- Focus on the muscle group being used.

Here's What I Want You to Add to Your Program
- Add two fifteen-minute weightlifting sessions a week (use Covert's Home Weightlifting Program or design your own program).
- Cut back to three aerobic/cross-training sessions a week.
- Increase two of these sessions to thirty minutes.
- Do the third session for fifteen to twenty minutes, adding wind sprints.*

*Do not add wind sprints to your program until you can walk a mile in twenty minutes without getting out of breath. Do not add wind sprints to your program until you have been on an aerobic exercise program for at least four weeks.

And now . . . Let's put it all together

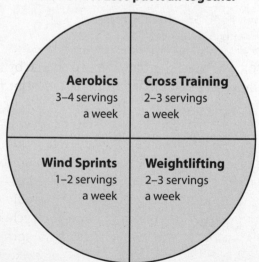

Aerobics	Cross Training
3–4 servings a week	2–3 servings a week
Wind Sprints	**Weightlifting**
1–2 servings a week	2–3 servings a week

24 The Four Food Groups of Exercise

Recommended Weekly Allowances

To get a balanced diet of exercise every week, you need to do something from each of the four exercise groups. You need to do lots of aerobics, some cross training, occasional wind sprints, and a little weightlifting. You may be thinking, "How am I ever going to find enough time to do all that?" Actually, it's simple because, just as if you were making dinner, you can make a "casserole" that contains a little bit from each of the four groups.

The main ingredient of your casserole is aerobic exercise. You need to do that three or four times a week, twenty to thirty minutes a session. To that you need to add cross training. Does that mean extra days, extra time? Luckily, no. Cross training is also aerobic exercise, isn't it? Pick two aerobic exercises, making one your main exercise and the other your cross-training exercise. Alternate the two so that by the end of the week you've done three or four aerobic sessions. In effect you've done aerobics and cross training, yet you haven't added any extra time to your exercise schedule.

Wind sprints should be done once a week, but here again you don't need to set aside a separate day to do them. They can be done during one of your aerobic sessions. Say you've chosen jogging and bicycling as your two aerobic exercises. You jog on Monday and Wednesday, and you cycle on Friday. All you have to do is add two to five wind sprints to one of those sessions — your Wednesday jog, for example. As a bonus, you can shorten your Wednesday workout by five to ten minutes, because the intensity of the added wind sprints allows you to reduce the total time you spend exercising.

Weightlifting is the only ingredient in the casserole that actually adds time to your exercise program. But it's not as time-consuming as you may think. You need to lift weights only a couple of times a week for fifteen to twenty-five minutes. You don't even need to work every muscle in each session; if you work a few of the bigger muscles, say by doing squats, push-ups, and sit-ups, you'll get the postexercise metabolic response you need.

There's a final ingredient in our casserole — *rest*. Don't leave it out! People who are eager to get fast results often forgo their needed rest and recuperation. *Recovery is as important as exercise!* It's during your rest periods that all the "good stuff" happens; that's when your muscles grow and repair and, most important, when you grow more fat-burning enzymes.

Basic Program

This program is not designed to add lots of muscle or to lower fat dramatically, but it is the most time-efficient way to get fit and to preserve the fitness you already have.

Day of week	What to do	How long?
Monday	Aerobic exercise #1	30 min.
Tuesday	Weightlifting	15–25 min.
Wednesday	Rest	
Thursday	Aerobic exercise #1 (with wind sprints)	20 min.
Friday	Weightlifting	15–25 min.
Saturday	Aerobic exercise #2	30 min.
Sunday	Rest	

Sample Programs

As you progress from beginner to advanced, instead of increasing the time you spend exercising — increase the intensity!

Beginners and Those over Sixty, Pregnant, or Recovering from Illness

Day of week	What to do
Monday	Walk
Tuesday	Covert's Home Weightlifting, level 1, 1–2 sets for each muscle area
Wednesday	Rest
Thursday	Walk (add 1–3 jogs, 20–40 seconds each, during your walk)
Friday	Covert's Home Weightlifting (as described for Tuesday)
Saturday	Aerobic rider or stationary bicycle
Sunday	Rest

Intermediate

Day of week	What to do
Monday	Jog
Tuesday	Covert's Home Weightlifting, level 2, 2–3 sets for each muscle area
Wednesday	Rest
Thursday	Jog (add 2–4 runs, 20–40 seconds each, during your jog)
Friday	Covert's Home Weightlifting (as described for Tuesday)
Saturday	Rowing machine
Sunday	Rest

Advanced

Day of week	What to do
Monday	Run
Tuesday	Covert's Home Weightlifting, level 3, 3–4 sets for each muscle area
Wednesday	Rest
Thursday	Run (add 3–5 sprints, 20–40 seconds each, during your run)
Friday	Covert's Home Weightlifting (as described for Tuesday)
Saturday	Mountain biking
Sunday	Rest

For People Who Want to Speed Up the Program

My basic program (page 132) will induce a steady, moderate weight loss (if you're overweight) while raising your fitness to a healthful level. If you want to lose weight more quickly or reach a higher level of fitness, give this speeded-up program a try. Please! If you find that it makes you too tired, cut back! Remember, if you are not recovering from the exercise, you're defeating the whole purpose of the program.

The Speeded-Up Program

Day of week	What to do	How long?
Monday	Aerobic exercise #1*	45 min. or two 20–25-min. sessions (one in A.M. and one in P.M.)
Tuesday	Covert's Home Weightlifting, 3–4 sets for each muscle area, level 1, 2, or 3	20–30 min.
Wednesday	Aerobic exercise #2*	45 min. or two sessions (as described for Monday)
Thursday	Covert's Home Weightlifting (as described for Tuesday)	20–30 min.
Friday	Aerobic exercise #1* (with wind sprints)	30 min.
Saturday	Aerobic exercise #2*	45 min. or two sessions (as described for Monday)
Sunday	Rest	

* For rapid fat loss, select weight-bearing and/or whole-body exercises such as jogging, walking, hiking, aerobics classes, rowing, cross-country skiing, treadmill, aerobic rider, stair climber, ladder climber, cross-country ski machine, or rowing machine. Swimming, water aerobics, and stationary bicycling, although excellent for fitness, are not conducive to rapid fat loss.

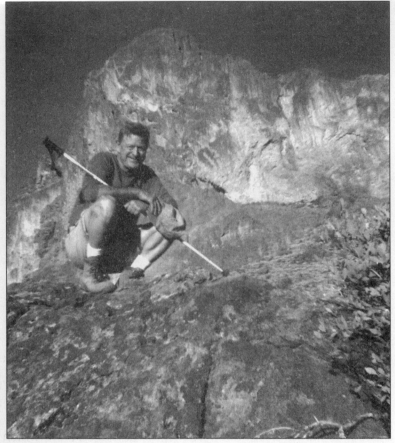

Michael Woods

I'm in training!
For what?
Oh, just training.
I'm thinking about
the mountains I'm going to climb,
the rivers yet to be paddled,
the square dance that lasts half the night.

— Covert Bailey, sixty-seven,
Superstition Mountains, Arizona, 1999

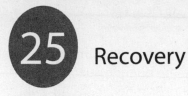

25 Recovery

If you scratch yourself, a protective scab forms to allow the skin to heal. When the scab falls off, the repaired skin looks just like new. After the redness goes away, you can't distinguish the new skin from the old. If you pull the scab off too soon, you delay the healing. Another scab forms, but this time the healing skin beneath the scab looks a little different. If you persistently pull off the scabs, you end up with scar tissue that's hard and rigid and doesn't look anything like the surrounding skin. It *feels* as if it's tougher, but as any physician will tell you, scar tissue is actually weaker than regular skin.

When you exercise, you damage your muscles. They, too, need time to repair. If you don't let them heal properly, they, like scar tissue, become weaker in a sense. But! If you allow them time to recover, the repaired muscles will be even stronger than they were before. Unlike damaged skin, which in healing seeks to imitate the previous skin, muscle tissue gets stronger and bigger and grows more fat-burning enzymes. It does everything it can to better withstand the stress of your next exercise session.

The obvious question is, how long do muscles need to recover? For weightlifting, recovery time is well defined. You need to rest for forty-eight hours between sessions. A famous female body builder tells the story of the problem she had developing her biceps. She worked her arms every day but

> **Exercise is worthless if you don't recover from it!**

saw no improvement. She increased the weights — with no better results. Finally, in frustration, she dropped back to lighter weights and lifted only every other day. Her poor muscles, finally getting a chance to repair, grew larger. Serious body builders don't ignore the forty-eight-hour rule. They know that all their hard work is worthless if they don't give their muscles time to repair. Some body builders lift every day, but they're careful to not use the same muscles each time. They might work the upper body one day, the lower body the next.

The amount of recovery time needed after aerobic exercise isn't so clear-cut. We say that twenty-four hours is usually sufficient, but that number varies with how old you are, how hard you exercised, and how long you did it. I don't think this issue requires a lot of discussion. Use your common sense. If you had a particularly hard or long exercise session, then wait longer before the next one. If you're older, allow more time for recovery. Do a greater variety of activities so that, like the body builders, you use different muscles.

Suppose that in your eagerness to get fit, you exercise too hard, too often, too long. You keep "pulling off the scab" before the muscles have time to repair. Well, muscles don't form scar tissue, but the body has other ways to signal you to slow down. One of the first signs is an increase in the resting heart rate. Normal resting heart rate is around seventy-two beats a minute, or even lower in fit people. When fatigue sets in from too much exercise, your resting heart rate goes up by ten or more beats per minute. If your resting pulse is higher than usual, take the day off or do a gentler workout.

A rise in blood pressure is another early indicator of muscle fatigue. Normal blood pressure is 120/80. When muscles don't get enough time to recuperate, the diastolic pressure (the bottom number) goes up.

If you stubbornly persist, continuing to exercise so hard or so often that the muscles never have time to recover, other symptoms will crop up. You may get diarrhea, you may sleep poorly, you may have a poor appetite. You may get cranky, depressed, or apathetic. If you still don't slow down, the muscles will finally give up and refuse to do their job. Your performance will drop off, and your muscles may even begin to atrophy.

I'll admit that I'm not good at following my own advice. I like to hike for hours and hours — really trash myself. And then I do it again the next day and the next. After a long, hard hike, I say to my muscles, "There! Let's see if you can fix that before tomorrow!" I think it's good to challenge yourself now and then, to exercise harder than usual. But! I don't persist for weeks on end. After two or three days of hard hiking, I give my muscles two or three days to recuperate.

It is foolish to challenge yourself endlessly while ignoring the warning signals. Some people are so addicted to exercise that they convince themselves all the symptoms of fatigue are normal, even healthful. You probably won't believe this, but an article was published once that said getting diarrhea as a result of exercise was a good sign because it meant the body was ridding itself of toxins! Great. If that's true, I pity the superfit athletes.

Given half a chance, your muscles will keep up with whatever exercise you give them. But pay attention when they need a break! If you are experiencing four or five of the symptoms listed on page 140, slow down, take a few days off, and allow more time between exercise sessions.

Symptoms Associated with Overexercising

Poor coordination
Slower reaction time
Sleep problems
Loss of appetite
Irritability
Diarrhea
Fatigue, lethargy
Muscle pain

Higher resting heart rate
Depression, apathy
Impaired performance
Joint pain
Weight loss, drawnappearance
Friends tell you that you are
   overdoing it
Heavy-legged feeling

26 Warming Up

Some people, impatient to get to their "real" exercise, neglect to warm up. They think they're just wasting time with a warm-up, that all the fat-burning and fitness improvements occur during the actual exercise. If you have a friend like that, give him this bit of information: exercise preceded by a warm-up launches the muscles into fat-burning *sooner* than exercise started at full bore. Your friend actually delays fat-burning if he doesn't warm up. He thinks he's saving time, but in reality he's getting fewer benefits from his exercise. If he doesn't believe you, ask him one simple question: "When you start your exercise without warming up, are you breathless for the first few minutes?" He'll probably admit that he is, and here's why.

The small capillaries that are woven around your muscles are collapsed when the muscles are cold. They don't open up until the muscle temperature rises. That means oxygen isn't delivered and fat isn't burned until you warm up.

If you start exercising at your usual aerobic pace, you are, in essence, running anaerobically for the first few minutes, because your cold muscles lack oxygen. Hence that breathlessness you experience.

> Warm muscles have a larger blood supply than cold muscles and therefore have more oxygen.

Your heart is also a muscle. You might not think it needs to be warmed up, since it beats all the time, but an exercising heart rate is double the resting heart rate. You wouldn't shift your car from first to fourth gear without going through second and third. Why do it to your body?

Cold muscles become more elastic, more stretchable as they warm up, so you're less likely to hurt yourself. And cold muscles mean cold nerves, so you don't have the coordination needed for running, jumping, or swerving during exercise. Cold muscles, cold nerves — you're asking for injury.

Warming Up!
- Increases blood flow to the muscles, which
- Brings more oxygen to the muscles, so that
- Enzymes can burn fat more quickly, which means
- You burn more fat!

The harder the upcoming exercise, the longer the warm-up should be. That rule doesn't need much explanation. If you're going to run a race, you need to warm up for fifteen minutes or more. A thirty-minute jog needs only about a five-minute warm-up. If your exercise is brisk walking, you may think you don't need to bother warming up, but even you should start at a slightly slower pace to warm your heart, muscles, and nerves.

A warm-up can be simply a gentler version of the upcoming exercise. Walk before a jog; jog before a run. Pedal more slowly than usual on your bicycle. Swim slowly, row slowly, ski slowly. Warm up at a pace that gets your heart beating at 50–60 percent of maximum (as compared to 65–80 percent of maximum during actual exercise). You should be breathing harder than normal but not as hard as during the actual exercise.

If your sport involves using specific muscles, expand your

warm-up to include these muscles. If you lift weights, for example, warm up your entire body first (as described above), then warm up individual muscles by using lighter weights for your first set of lifts. If you're a baseball pitcher or a tennis player, warm the muscles in your arm by doing several fake throws or swings, slowly and gently.

27 Spot Reducing

Next to quick weight-loss diets, spot reducing has to be the biggest rip-off foisted on the American public. Most of us laugh at those old-fashioned bumping and rolling devices that were supposed to jiggle the fat away. But I'll bet almost every woman has been suckered into doing leg lifts to get rid of thigh fat, and every man has done sit-ups to work off his belly fat. I'm as guilty as anyone. I was starting to get a little roll around my midsection, so I did sit-ups. In the morning, in the afternoon, in the evening. I did more than three hundred sit-ups a day! My abdominal muscles got hard as a rock, but the fat on top never moved. My belly felt like Jell-O on top of a washboard.

Let me say it loud and clear. YOU CANNOT SPOT-REDUCE! You can't work a specific muscle with the idea that the fat on top of the muscle will be burned off. Just because fat tends to collect in specific areas doesn't mean working that area is going to dislodge it. In women, fat tends to be deposited in the upper thighs and buttocks; in men, it collects in the belly. But the fat doesn't "belong" to those areas. Exercising those muscles to lose the fat in those areas is silly.

Fat is like blood. If you cut your finger, you don't get finger blood. You get blood. The fat on your thighs isn't thigh fat — it's fat! The fat on your belly isn't belly fat — it's fat! Fat "belongs" to your entire body, to be used wherever and whenever it's needed for fuel. When you jog, your muscles don't say, "Oh! She's jogging, we'll use her leg fat." They say, "Send me some fat—any kind, from anywhere."

It makes sense, then, that if you want to lose a lot of fat, you need to use a lot of muscles. Using one small muscle to get rid of pounds of fat is ludicrous. The abdominal muscles resemble a dinner plate in size and shape. When men do sit-ups to get rid of belly fat, they're asking a small set of muscles to handle a big load. Such small muscles just aren't big enough to burn much fat. Similarly, women try to get rid of the fat on their thighs by doing leg raises, which use the outer thigh muscles. Compared to the big quadriceps muscles on the front of the thighs, the muscles on the outside of the thighs are very small. When worked, they don't burn much fat. Exercising only one muscle or a relatively small set of muscles doesn't use many calories. But when you exercise large sets of muscles, fat is drawn from all parts of the body to meet the energy requirements. It follows that to get rid of fat, be it belly fat or thigh fat, you must use your biggest, hungriest (calorie-consuming) muscles. Stop doing sit-ups and leg raises, get up off the floor, and use the largest muscles in your body, the ones in your thighs and buttocks—the very muscles used in all aerobic exercise.

You may argue that spot reducing works because you've been doing leg raises for years and now your legs appear much slimmer. Actually, the leg raises have made the *muscles* in your legs firmer, so the area looks less fat. You increased muscle rather than losing fat. The *only* way to burn fat off your thighs is to do whole-body, gentle aerobic exercise.

> To burn off fat — use your biggest and hungriest muscles — the more the better!

Let me emphasize again that fat belongs to the WHOLE body. Once they

> If spot reducing worked, people who chew gum would have skinny faces!

understand that fact, most people accept the idea that the fat in their bellies and thighs will be burned off more readily with large-muscle buttocks and thigh exercises than with sit-ups or leg raises. But as the fat slowly creeps upward into the arms and the neck, it gets harder to imagine that a *lower-body* exercise can treat an *upper-body* problem. It's easy to get suckered into doing spot-reducing exercises for these areas. When our arms seem too fleshy, we flap them about like land-bound birds. To smooth out a double chin, we contort our faces into clown smiles while trying to touch our noses with our tongues. Believe me, it won't work. When fat appears in your upper body, it is merely an indication that you've "topped off" the lower body fat. The cure is the same. Get on your feet and use the biggest, hungriest muscles you've got!

You could, of course, resort to drastic measures to spot-reduce. Try putting your arm in a cast for several months. When you take the cast off, that arm will definitely be smaller, because you lose muscle as the tissue atrophies. Theoretically, a woman with large thighs who was willing to do anything to reduce their bulk could have casts put on her legs until they wasted away. Unfortunately, she wouldn't lose *fat* from her thighs because fat doesn't atrophy—muscle does. In fact, while her legs were in those casts losing muscle, the fat in her thighs would increase. Not a very healthy or practical thing to do.

Are spot-reducing exercises worthless? Not at all! In fact, I highly recommend them—they are great for spot *building!* I don't criticize the exercises; I criticize the people who label them spot reducing. Spot reducing, after all, is actually a mild form of weightlifting. The "burn" you feel during these exercises is an indication that you're building muscle rather than burning fat. Take advantage of that! You can enhance the shape of your body by emphasizing a particular area, thus making the surrounding areas appear slimmer.

A woman who came to my clinic achieved a dramatic change in her body shape by spot building. For years, she had struggled with her "milk-bottle" figure, doing lots and lots of spot-reducing exercises for her hips and thighs. All that did was make her lower body bigger, not slimmer. Once she realized that spot reducing was actually spot *building*, she changed her focus and exercised to get bigger in the right places. She did lots of aerobic exercise to slim her lower body and did upper-body weightlifting to fill out her upper body. The milk-bottle look disappeared.

I'm not against spot-reducing exercises. I just want you to get your head on straight about what they really do. They shape muscle; they do not burn fat. They build; they don't reduce. One reason I like aerobics classes is that they combine fat-burning aerobic exercises and "spot-reducing" exercises so well. For part of the hour you're on your feet burning off fat, then you're on the floor doing muscle-firming work. If you prefer to call the floor work spot reducing instead of gentle weightlifting, that's okay — as long as you realize that you're firming the muscle, not reducing the fat.

I can't let a discussion of spot reducing end without some comments on cellulite. Cellulite is just plain fat deposited in areas where the skin and underlying support tissue tend to pucker and wrinkle. It isn't a special kind of fat but rather a special kind of skin *over* the fat. Have you noticed that some very fat women do not have cellulite? A woman can have very large legs that jiggle when she walks, yet her skin may be smooth and unwrinkled. Obviously, the wrinkled, puckered look of cellulite is not a measure of the quantity of fat in the legs. In fact, we sometimes see very thin women with lots of cellulite. The conclusion: cellulite is wrinkly skin, which, like stretch marks and scars, shows more on some women than on others.

If you have cellulite, think not of losing fat but rather of tightening skin. Just as you pull up sagging pantyhose, you can also pull up the tops of your thighs and find that suddenly the cellulite is gone. A good way to tighten your skin is to build up the muscle underneath. I explained earlier that hamstring exercises and leg lifts *do not* spot reduce, but they DO bulk up muscle, which makes the skin more taut, thus helping to make the cellulite less obvious.

28 Golf and Other
Subaerobic Exercises

Those of us in the fitness field like to make fun of golf, treating it as nonexercise, an activity that keeps your heart rate way below the magical 65–80 percent of maximum. And yet eighteen holes of golf (not using a cart) leaves one feeling pleasantly tired, glad to put the feet up. Clearly, something good has resulted from this exercise, even though golf is not aerobic. Common sense tells us that golf and other such low-intensity activities have value even though they aren't included in the tables of "good" exercise.

I use the term "subaerobic" for low-intensity pursuits that aren't intense enough to be aerobic yet that still involve some effort. If you were to take your heart rate during subaerobic exercise, it would be between 50 and 65 percent of maximum. That's not enough to make you breathe deeply, but if you do the activity long enough, your body warms up and you feel that you've gotten some exercise. And you DO get aerobic benefits from golf or any low-intensity exercise — you just have to do a lot of it! I have a friend who never exercises aerobically. He never does anything that makes him breathe deeply. All he does is walk. Day after day, week after week, year after year. His blood pressure is low, his cholesterol is low, he's lean and healthy. He's a postman, and he's very fit.

I believe the reason we don't hear as much about the benefits of subaerobic exercise is that the studies required to measure them would take too long. If we got a thousand people together and had them do aerobic exercise, we'd see measurable improvements in six months. We'd be able to demonstrate that their fat-burning enzymes increased and their cholesterol level and blood pressure were lowered. But suppose we got one thousand people to do subaerobic exercise—got all one thousand of them traipsing behind my postman friend. We would have to study them for years before we could show beneficial results.

It's the quick results that give aerobic exercise such good press. When people exercise hard enough to get their heart rates in that range of 65–80 percent of maximum, then *everyone* shows improvement in a matter of months. Not some people, *everybody*. And that's incredible. No matter what their prior condition, aerobic exercise makes everyone healthier in short order. Subaerobic exercise has the same effect on our bodies, but it takes much longer.

Very fit peopie have the distinct advantage of making subaerobic exercise into play. A game of Frisbee, for example, is subaerobic play for fit kids, while their fat parents sit and watch. If the fat parents join the "fun," they are not exercising subaerobically — they are aerobic, with their pulses in the 65–80 percent zone. Or the parents may be so out of shape that playing Frisbee with the kids makes them out-of-breath anaerobic.

The point is that fit people get the benefits of subaerobic exercise when they are playing, not thinking about exercise at all. If they add "real" exercise, their exercise total can be substantial. I can't emphasize this point enough. Once you get fit, activities that used to seem like exercise work become play, so you can do lots of it.

If you are overweight and/or unfit, my constant harping on the benefits of exercise and my constant pushing to do a

The Zones of Exercise

	Subaerobic	Aerobic	Anaerobic
Heart rate	50%–65% of maximum	65%–80% of maximum	80%–100% of maximum
Perceived level of exertion	Easy to moderate	Somewhat hard	Hard
Breathing Talking	Moderate Can talk comfortably	Deep Can talk haltingly	Gasping Can't talk
Fat burned during exercise	The total of calories burned is low, but a high percentage of them are fat.	The total of calories burned is moderate to high, and a moderate to high percentage of them are fat.	The total of calories burned is high, but a very low percentage of them are fat.
Growth of fat-burning enzymes after exercise	Low to moderate increase	High increase	Moderate increase
Fitness-increasing capabilities	Low to moderate	Moderate to high	High
Covert's comments	As you get fitter, exercises that used to be hard become easy, so more and more of your activities become subaerobic.	The most efficient zone of exercise, with the most benefits for the least amount of time.	Competitive athletes must train often in this zone; occasional anaerobic exercise improves the fitness of the average person.

lot of it may seem overwhelming. To keep yourself going, think about young, healthy kids, playing Frisbee and volleyball, running and biking. They do those things as play after they come home from school sports. The average kid doesn't *have* an exercise program. When you get fit, you won't either.

You won't ask if you should do twenty minutes of this exercise or fifteen minutes of that one. You will get more exercise from playing volleyball in the afternoon and line dancing in the evening than you do now from a formal exercise program.

So! Aerobic exercise is not the only way to get fit. If we could live our lives doing subaerobic exercise *all the time*, we wouldn't need to talk about aerobics so much.

29 The Body Has a Plan!

Exercise is stressful. It tears up muscles, pounds bones, drives up blood pressure (during the exercise), raises body temperature, and produces all kinds of noxious waste products. After you get through jogging for a half hour, your body doesn't say, "Whoopee! That was great!" It groans and starts to clean up the mess.

Think about that amazing fact! Your car doesn't repair itself. Cat scratches on your favorite chair don't go away by themselves. Only living things have the ability to self-heal and sometimes be even better after the injury than before. Your body has a plan—it repairs itself!! After you exercise it becomes stronger, better able to withstand the stress the next time you exercise. It makes you tougher. In the same way your hands form tough calluses if you hoe a lot of weeds, your body becomes tougher, both physically and mentally, from the stress of exercise.

The more you exercise, the more adaptations your body makes. As you get fitter, your body adapts more and more, so exercise becomes less and less stressful.

The body's plan is simple. "Nobody is going to get the best of me! I'm going to use my internal defense mechanisms to fight off any insult. Bring on the bacte-

> Fit people are tough! Tough enough to benefit from the stress of exercise.

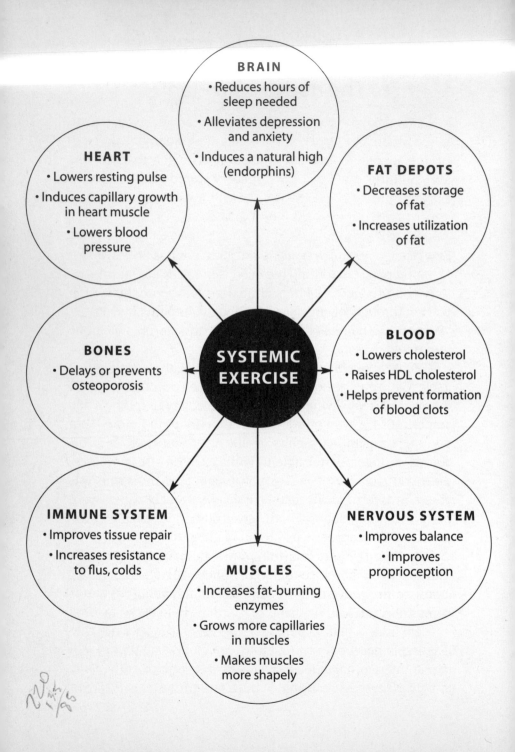

ria — I have white blood cells. Bring on the scratches and burns — I will make new skin. Damage my bones — I will build stronger ones! I have an emergency plan for every tissue, every organ, every cell of my being. If you damage any part of me, I will repair and rebuild it stronger than it was. Weightlifting? Ha! I will expend every stored calorie I have to put my muscle right. Running? Easy! My master has stored excess calories these many years, and I will use them to rebuild, repair, and make me stronger inside than ever. Fat, stored on hips, packed on midsections — I will use it all in my efforts to prepare for the next insult."

Losing fat has been the main focus of this book, but to your body, burning fat is no more than an expedient way to accomplish its REAL goal — improving your health. Fat loss is just icing on the cake. I'll be honest with you. I've used the title *Fit or Fat* all these years because it's an attention-grabber. I could have titled this book *The Change-Your-Whole-Body Fitness Program,* but you wouldn't have bought it. I could fill pages and pages with all the benefits of aerobic exercise — but you'd be out buying the latest diet book instead.

Take a look at the diagram on page 154. Aerobic, systemic, whole-body exercise affects every tissue, every organ in the body. I'm not going to bore you by describing every change that happens when you exercise. We've all heard that exercise makes the heart and lungs healthier. But there are quirky little benefits you may never have heard about. For example, you'd be wise to ride in vehicles driven by fit people because they have better coordination and ability to handle stressful situations, so they are more likely to avoid automobile accidents. And if you plan on getting old, you'd be smart to keep fit because exercise makes your blood thinner so your aging heart can pump it more easily. If you're anticipating minor surgery, start exercising, because fit tissues heal more quickly. And this sounds like a bad joke, but fit smokers fare better than unfit smokers. Even the bad things we do to ourselves are lessened by the good things exercise does for us.

I focus on fat because that's the one symptom of poor fitness that everyone can recognize. How many books would sell with the title *Being Fit Makes Your Liver Healthy?* How many people would be out exercising if I went on talk shows raving about the effects of aerobics on blood chemistry?

I can sympathize with the frustration of physicians who wish that their patients would exercise, for doctors know their patients' problems would be less or even nonexistent if they had exercised in the past. Telling a man that exercise helps keep blood cholesterol in line doesn't register until he has a heart attack. Discussions relating exercise to insulin levels are boring—until you get diabetes. Talks about the effects of exercise on bone density don't hit home — until you get "old lady's broken hip" from osteoporosis.

But everybody talks about fat. You can see it, pinch it, weigh it, and hate it. People listen to fat talk! So for all those doctors out there who can't get patients motivated to improve their systemic health, try this. Tell your patients, "If you get fit, you won't be fat." They will listen. Period. End of discussion.

Questions about the
Four Food Groups of Exercise

Q: **You say I should exercise for twenty to thirty minutes.
What should I do if I can't last for twenty minutes?**

A: If you can't do your exercise because you get out of
breath, you've either selected an exercise that is too difficult for you or you're exercising too hard. Find an easier
exercise or *slow down!* Now if you're really out of shape, it
may be hard for you to do ANY exercise for twenty minutes nonstop because your legs and feet get tired. If that
happens, shorten your exercise session to ten minutes
and do it twice a day. Each week add an extra minute or
two until you can do twenty minutes without stopping.

Q: **Is swimming a good cross-training sport?**

A: Yes, one of the best. However, be cautious in the beginning — it's hard to know if you're aerobic when you swim.
Breathing isn't an accurate monitor for beginners because
they usually can't get enough air, and it's not that easy to
take your pulse. If you do take your pulse, be aware that
your heart rate in the water is about ten beats slower than
on land. The horizontal position you assume when swimming and the cooling effect of the water lower your heart
rate. You have to adjust your training heart rate ten beats
downward. Since both breathing and heart rate are hard
to monitor when you swim, remember to take it easy in
the beginning. Find a pace that's comfortable so you can
swim for twenty minutes or longer.

Q: **You always talk about sprinting during a walk or a jog. Is that the ONLY way to do wind sprints?**

A: You can do a sprint during ANY aerobic exercise. You can bicycle faster, swim faster, row faster, whatever. Keep in mind also that you can sprint by increasing the resistance of the exercise. A hill in the middle of your run offers increased resistance; you don't have to speed up at all to get the wind-sprint effect. Similarly, you can increase the resistance on a stationary bicycle or raise the incline on a treadmill to get the wind-sprint effect.

Q: **Why do wind sprints make me so tired?**

A: The first day you add wind sprints to your exercise, you probably will feel more fatigued. That's why I have you shorten your exercise on that day by five to ten minutes. But if you're really exhausted, then you're probably doing your wind sprints too hard or too long. Remember, speed up just a little bit and sprint for just a few seconds. If you take your pulse, it should be only ten to fifteen beats faster than your aerobic pulse. The most important thing about wind sprinting is not the sprint itself but your ability to recover after it. If you're very fat, go for a brisk walk and do a ten- to twenty-second "shuffle walk" in the middle. The purpose is not to exhaust yourself but to train your body to get back to an aerobic level while recovering from a mild increase in intensity.

Q: **Will I get even fitter if I do wind sprints during every aerobic session?**

A: Yes, I suppose so, but why do the same thing day after day? You will get bored, quit exercising, and rip this book into tiny pieces. Kidding aside, your question misses the point. You should do a lot of aerobic exercise, a *whole* lot — whenever you can, as often as you can — and put a little hill in the middle of your walk or jog so that nobody knows you are doing a wind sprint, not even you. Get fit the natural way.

Q: Is there any exercise that will help me lose my cellulite?

A: Yes, sometimes weightlifting can help. If you build up the muscles in an area, the skin on top of those muscles may smooth out. Fat under the skin looks lumpy, but muscle under the skin looks smooth.

The classic place to find cellulite is in the back of the upper leg, and one of the best exercises to smooth out this area is the hamstring curl. Special machines for this exercise can be found in most weightlifting facilities. Lie on your stomach, insert your ankles under a roller bar, and pull upward with your legs until your ankles almost touch your buttocks. At home you can take the same position on the floor while someone puts resistance on your legs by gently pulling back on your ankles as you pull up toward your buttocks.

I stressed earlier that cellulite is *not* a fat problem but a skin problem. It's not a "special" fat, as some people would have you believe. It's just plain old fat bulging out under skin that has lost some of its elasticity. Cellulite is more apparent in older women, especially those with fair skin. Women who go to plastic surgeons to have their cellulite removed are sometimes disappointed with the results because their fat was helping to keep the skin taut. Once the fat is suctioned out, the skin that covered it may be even looser, so it dimples and puckers even more. Plastic surgeons know that liposuction works best on people whose skin is still elastic and tight. If you have cellulite and choose to lose fat the natural way, with exercise, be sure to couple it with muscle-building exercises to keep the skin as taut as possible.

Q: **I was about sixty pounds overweight. I lost weight pretty quickly when I first started your program, but once I added the weightlifting component, my weight loss seemed to stop. Now I'm stuck with forty more pounds to lose. What should I do?**

A: Occasionally, very overweight people are discouraged when weightlifting is added to their weight-loss program. These individuals' muscles seem to bulk up quite readily, so their weightlifting is adding muscle weight. Even though they are losing fat, their weight doesn't drop as fast as they expected. If you're one of these individuals, that is, if you sense you're getting much stronger very quickly but not losing weight, consider dropping the weightlifting part until you're within twenty pounds of your desired weight.

Q: **I'm a five-foot-four woman who weighs 180 pounds. When I calculated my lean body mass the result was 120, much higher than the LBMs shown in your table (Chapter 7). With that much lean, your formula projects an ideal weight of 154 pounds, which seems much too heavy for my height.**

A: Sometimes the lean body mass of a person who is quite overweight is greater than normal. That's because her muscles have enlarged to carry around the excess weight. Ideally, an overweight person should try to retain as much muscle as possible while losing weight because it is muscle that burns up the calories she eats. But, realistically, most people who need to lose more than twenty-five pounds find they can't avoid losing some muscle; when your weight drops, your muscles have a lighter load to carry and thus don't need to be as large as they were. After you've shed some of your weight, recalculate your lean body mass. You'll find that it is smaller and that your projected ideal weight will be lower.

Q: **Is there a best time to exercise?**

A: Yes! You should exercise precisely at 1:32 P.M. every day. I'm joking, of course. Research has shown that more Olympic medals have been won between 1 and 2 P.M. than at any other time, so some fools think that's when you should exercise. Pretty silly. As I said earlier, the best time to exercise is whenever you'll *do* it. Some people are morning people, full of energy and raring to go at an early hour. Other people like to exercise after work to ease the tensions of the day. I'm retired now, so I exercise any time I feel like it. Exercise physiologists tell us that morning exercisers tend to stick with their programs more consistently than afternoon exercisers. But tests on the afternoon exercisers indicate that they have a higher tolerance to stress. So take your pick: you can be an uptight morning exerciser who never falls off the wagon, or you can be a relaxed, on-again-off-again afternoon exerciser.

Q: **I'm one of those older guys you wrote about who exercise a lot, and I'm losing upper-body muscle. What should I do?**

A: As you get older, your body's ability to repair itself decreases, so ALL your muscles tend to atrophy. Suppose you put the left arm of a twenty-year-old and that of a seventy-year-old in casts for two months. At the end of that time the seventy-year-old's arm would be much more wasted than the twenty-year-old's. Young people have a natural resistance to losing muscle.

If you had the twenty-year-old pedal a stationary bicycle for four hours a day, five days a week, in six months he'd have rock-hard legs, and his upper body would look pretty much the same as before. Not so with the seventy-year-old. His leg muscles would be strong, but the muscles in his upper body would slowly atrophy. It's as if his body were saying, "I *have* to repair the leg muscles because he uses them so much, but at my age, I can't waste time on the arm and chest muscles."

So you have to USE your upper body if you want to keep your muscle. The obvious thing to do is lift weights, working your shoulder, back, chest, and arm muscles. Then let them rest for at least forty-eight hours before you do it again. Remember that exercise is not effective if you don't allow your body time to recuperate from it.

You could also do an aerobic exercise that has an upper-body component, such as rowing or swimming. Or you could incorporate muscle-building activities into your playtime. I jog or bicycle every day for fitness, but I do archery and rock climbing for fun. Those sports really work the upper body. I enjoy them so much that I don't think of them as "weightlifting," even though they are.

Q: **I'm only 22 percent fat, but my thighs jiggle! My husband has a big belly, but it doesn't jiggle at all!**

A: Women often complain, "No matter what I do, I can't get rid of my jiggly thighs!" At 22 percent fat (considered a healthful level for women), most women still have fat in their thighs. It jiggles because it builds up right under the skin. In contrast, abdominal fat in men initially accumulates beneath the abdominal muscles. A man's belly may be fat, but it doesn't jiggle because the muscles are stretched taut over the fat. Women's thighs usually stop jiggling when total fat gets down to 18 percent, but I've seen women who have as little as 15 percent fat (exceptionally low for women) and whose bodies look too thin — yet their thighs still jiggle. I'm sorry if this sounds sexist, but women's breasts jiggle also. Jiggly thighs in women are NORMAL. That's part of being female.

Q: **Hey Covert, have you thrown out YOUR bathroom scale?**

A: I've told many an audience, "Throw out your bathroom scales! Get body fat tested instead." No, I haven't thrown mine out. In fact, I have a very good bathroom scale that is as accurate as the one in a doctor's office. I step on it from time to time, but I don't make the mistake of thinking that every weight fluctuation is a change in body fat. If I lose a pound from one morning to the next, I think about what that pound might have been. Did I perhaps exercise in the sun without replacing fluids? Or if I've lost a pound or two in the space of a week, is it muscle loss because I haven't kept up my home weightlifting routine? If I were an older woman and seemed to lose weight continuously over months or a year, I would have to consider whether it was bone loss. So! My exhortation to throw away your bathroom scale is really for people who refuse to think about these subtle things. In fact, a scale is a wonderful tool if you don't assume that it weighs *fat*.

Q: **Are there other ways to know if I'm losing fat?**

A: One of the simplest ways to know if you're losing fat is to take your measurements. A pound of muscle takes up less space than a pound of fat. Exercise helps you lose fat — but it also helps you gain muscle. If you're *losing* fat but *gaining* muscle, you may not lose any weight at all. But you should notice a decrease in clothing size as slim muscle replaces bulky fat. Men — you carry most of your fat in your belly; the quickest way to know if you're losing fat is to measure your waistline every month or so. Women — measure your thighs and buttocks to see if your fat is shrinking.

Q: Are the body fat percentages (15 percent for men and 22 percent for women) the absolute highest one can be and still be healthy?

A: The percentages are not absolutes; the correct percentage for your body varies quite a lot with age and genetic makeup. The fat percentage number is really a comparison of lean weight (muscle and bone) to fat weight. If the lean weight is low because the person's bones are light, then the fat percentage is artificially increased. I say "artificially" because the actual pounds of body fat may not be high, but if there is less bone in proportion to the fat, the *percentage* of fat goes up.

Asian people, for example, have light, porous bones, so the recommended percentages are too low. For them, 18 percent for men and 25 percent for women are healthful levels. Black people usually have heavier, denser bones, and their healthful fat levels are 12 percent for men and 19 percent for women.

Female hormones also affect body fat; birth control pills raise the fat percentage somewhat, and hormone replacement therapy (for menopausal symptoms) seems to raise it even more. Bone loss in older women will also artificially raise the fat percentage.

Men have much less excuse for deviating from 15 percent (or 12 percent for blacks, 18 percent for Asians). They can't blame a fat gain on hormones or childbearing. And bone loss isn't as large an issue with men until they are well into their eighties.

Q: Which aerobic exercise is the very best?

A: It's true that I push some aerobic exercises more than others. For example, I think aerobic riders are far better than stationary bicycles because they use more muscles and have a whole-body effect. I tell people not to use swimming as their only exercise if they want to lose fat, but I encourage swimming for people who have injuries or arthritis and for pregnant women. In general, I prefer outdoor exercises to indoor machines. Not all aerobic exercises are created equal. Some build muscle more easily (rowing, bicycling), while others burn fat more easily (jogging, cross-country skiing). Some make you fit in a short time but have a high risk of injury (running, jumping rope), while others are very safe but also burn fat very slowly (swimming, water aerobics). The most important thing is to pick an exercise you like so that you will do a lot of it. The very best aerobic exercise is the one you will do.

Let me tell you what it's like to write a book. You create what you think is perfection. You send it to your editor. It comes back with so many red-marked corrections that you feel as if you were back in third grade.

In 1978, when I wrote the first edition of *Fit or Fat?* I didn't like those red marks because I thought they represented criticism of my writing. Now they make me smile. My editors grasp my meanings better than I do. When they suggest a different word or phrase, it enhances rather than distorts. I find myself thinking, "Yes! That's exactly what I wanted to say."

And who does all this? It's a team of people, really, but in that team there is a special person, a quiet, unassuming woman who scrutinizes my writing, each and every word. She's like a ghost to me because I've never met her face to face, but her fine touch surely has saved my books from extinction. Thank you, thank you, thank you, Peg Anderson.

And years ago, before Peg Anderson joined the team, there was Ruth Hapgood, who started it all. Thank you, Ruth, for taking a chance with me when I was unknown. And for letting me use the title *Fit or Fat?* when all my friends insisted it would never sell.

Index